Lymphoma Unlocked

With Orthodox and Alternative Treatment

Preface

I have written this book so that the patients suffering from Lymphoma can understand the disease in detail and choose a suitable treatment for them. This book provides simple approach about the clinical symptoms, complications, diagnosis, staging and treatments. In the last 15 years there has been considerable research and progress in the field of clinical studies, etiology, pathology, diagnosis and treatment of Lymphoma.

In this book, I have written in detail about Orthodox and Alternative Treatment (Budwig Protocol, which is the best alternative treatment and gives authentic success). Patient can carefully select the right treatment for him. This book has up to date information.

Dr. O.P.Verma

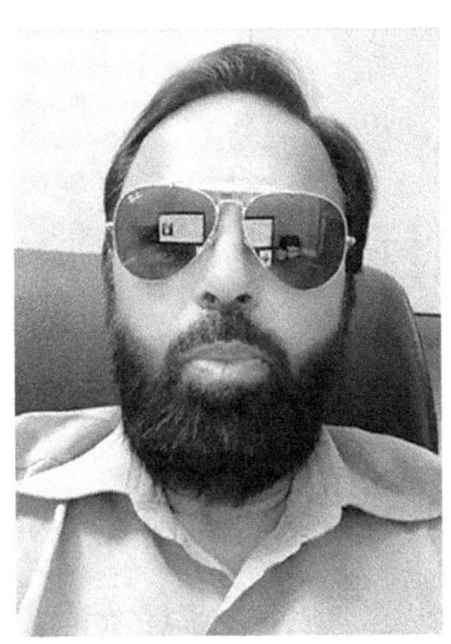

Written by
Dr. O.P.Verma
M.B.B.S., M.R.S.H. (London)
Budwig Wellness
7-B-43, Mahaveer Nagar III, Kota (Raj.)
https://gobudwig.com
+919460816360

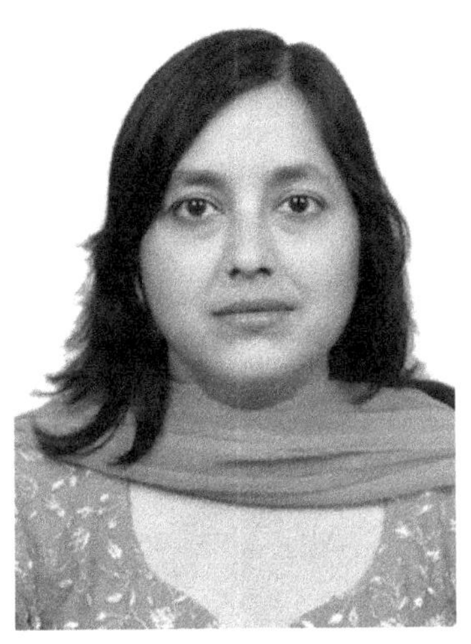

Edited by
Aishvarya Sharma
Senior Manager
Software A.G.
Bengaluru, Karnataka
B.Tech., I.I.T. B.H.U., Varanasi U.P.

Table of Content

LYMPHATIC SYSTEM - STRUCTURE AND FUNCTION 1

    LYMPH AND LYMPH VESSELS 2
    LYMPH NODES 2
    SPLEEN AND THYMUS 3
    LYMPHOCYTES 3
    FUNCTIONS OF LYMPHOCYTES 5

LYMPHOMA 6

    HODGKIN LYMPHOMA 6
    NON-HODGKIN LYMPHOMA (NHL) 6

NON-HODGKIN LYMPHOMA (NHL) 8

STATISTICS 9

RISK FACTORS OF LYMPHOMA 11

    COMMON RISK FACTORS 11
    AGE 12
    SEX 12
    IMMUNE DYSFUNCTION 13
    GENETICS 13
    INFECTIONS 15
    ENVIRONMENTAL TOXINS 16
    CANCER THERAPY 16
    LIFESTYLE FACTORS 17
    OBESITY 17
    BREAST IMPLANTS 18

TYPES OF NHL 19

    INDOLENT NHL 20
    AGGRESSIVE NHL 20
    DIFFUSE LARGE B-CELL LYMPHOMA (DLBCL) 21
    FOLLICULAR LYMPHOMA 22
    MANTLE CELL LYMPHOMA 23
    SMALL LYMPHOCYTIC LYMPHOMA 24
    DOUBLE HIT/TRIPLE HIT LYMPHOMA 24
    PRIMARY MEDIASTINAL LARGE B-CELL LYMPHOMA 24
    SPLENIC MARGINAL ZONE B-CELL LYMPHOMA 25
    EXTRANODAL MARGINAL ZONE B-CELL LYMPHOMA MALT 25

Nodal marginal zone B-cell lymphoma 26
Lymphoplasmacytic lymphoma 26
Primary effusion lymphoma 27
Burkitt lymphoma 27
Anaplastic large cell lymphoma, primary cutaneous 28
Anaplastic large cell lymphoma, systemic 29
Peripheral T-cell lymphoma 29
Angioimmunoblastic T-cell lymphoma 30
Adult T-cell lymphoma/leukemia 30
Extranodal NK/T-cell lymphoma, nasal type 31
Enteropathy-associated T-cell lymphoma 31
Hepatosplenic T-cell lymphoma 31
Subcutaneous panniculitis-like T-cell lymphoma 31
Mycosis fungoides 32

SYMPTOMS, AND COMPLICATIONS 33

Frequent Symptoms 33
Lymphadenopathy Types 34
Extranodal Symptoms 35
Primary extranodal lymphoma 36
Secondary extranodal lymphoma 36
Gastrointestinal Tract 36
Cutaneous (skin) lymphoma 37
Bone and Bone Marrow 37
Central Nervous System 38
Lungs 39
Liver 39
Kidneys and Adrenal Glands 40
Genitals 40
Complications 41
Cancer 41
Heart Disease 42
Hormonal Disorders and Infertility 42

DIAGNOSIS 44

Medical history and physical exam 44
Biopsy 44
Excisional or incisional biopsy 45
Needle biopsy 46
Bone marrow aspiration and biopsy 47

Lumbar puncture (spinal tap) 48
Pleural or peritoneal fluid sampling 48
Chromosome tests 50
Cytogenetics 50
Fluorescent in situ hybridization (FISH) 50
Imaging tests 51
Blood tests 54

NON-HODGKIN LYMPHOMA STAGES 56

Lugano classification 56
Stage I 57
Stage II 57
Stage III 57
Stage IV 58
How staging might affect treatment 58

DIFFERENTIAL DIAGNOSIS 59

NHL LYMPHOMA TREATMENT 60

Active Surveillance 60
Chemotherapy 61
Radiation Therapy 62
Chemotherapy 63
Alkylating agents 64
Corticosteroids 64
Platinum drugs 64
Anti-metabolites 64
Anthracyclines 64
Others 64
ABVD regimen 65
BEACOPP regimen 65
CHOP regimen 65
R-CHOP regimen 66
Possible side effects 66
Other drugs used to treat lymphoma 68
Immunotherapy for NHL 69
Monoclonal antibodies 69
Antibodies that target CD20 69
Rituximab (Rituxan) 70
Antibodies targeting CD52 71
Antibodies that target CD30 71

ANTIBODIES THAT TARGET CD79B 72
IMMUNE CHECKPOINT INHIBITORS 72
IMMUNOMODULATING DRUGS 72
CHIMERIC ANTIGEN RECEPTOR (CAR) T-CELL THERAPY 73
TARGETED THERAPY DRUGS FOR NHL 75
PROTEASOME INHIBITORS 75
HISTONE DEACETYLASE (HDAC) INHIBITORS 75
KINASE INHIBITORS 76
BRUTON'S TYROSINE KINASE (BTK) INHIBITORS 76
PI3K INHIBITORS 77
STEM CELL TRANSPLANT 78

PROGNOSIS **79**

HODGKIN LYMPHOMA **81**

DISCOVERY AND NOMENCLATURE HISTORY 81
INCIDENCE 82
RISK FACTORS 82
TYPES OF HODGKIN LYMPHOMA 84
CLASSIC HODGKIN LYMPHOMA (CHL) 84
NODULAR SCLEROSIS HODGKIN LYMPHOMA 85
LYMPHOCYTE-RICH CLASSIC HODGKIN LYMPHOMA 85
MIXED CELLULARITY HODGKIN LYMPHOMA 85
LYMPHOCYTE-DEPLETED HODGKIN LYMPHOMA 85
NODULAR LYMPHOCYTE-PREDOMINANT HODGKIN LYMPHOMA 86
SYMPTOMS 86
GENERAL SYMPTOMS 87
SPECIFIC SYMPTOMS 88

DIAGNOSIS **89**

STAGES **93**

PROGNOSTIC FACTORS **95**

TREATMENT HL 96
CHEMOTHERAPY 97
FIRST-LINE CHEMOTHERAPY 97
SECOND-LINE CHEMOTHERAPY 98
IMMUNOTHERAPY 100
MONOCLONAL ANTIBODIES 100
RADIATION 102
SIDE EFFECTS 102

STEM CELL TRANSPLANTS 103

ALTERNATIVE CANCER TREATMENTS **104**

LAETRILE (VITAMIN B-17) THERAPY...............................**106**

THE GERSON THERAPY **112**

SIMONCINI'S BAKING SODA CANCER TREATMENT **116**

BEST ALTERNATIVE TREATMENT - BUDWIG PROTOCOL...........**117**

PRIME CAUSE OF CANCER **121**

OTTO WARBURG – BIOGRAPHY 121
PRIME CAUSE OF CANCER 123

DR. JOHANNA BUDWIG - BIOGRAPHY & SCIENCE **125**

BUDWIG PROTOCOL..**132**

BUDWIG DIET...134
PRECAUTIONS...141
PROHIBITIONS OF BUDWIG PROTOCOL 144
FEW DESSERTS RECIPES BY DR. BUDWIG 146
ELDI OILS 148
COFFEE ENEMA 153
EPSOM BATH..155
SODA BICARB BATH..157
SUN THERAPY...157
HOW LONG SHOULD YOU TAKE THIS PROTOCOL? 158
LINOMEL 159
DAYLIGHT 159

DISCLAIMER **161**

MY BOOKS **162**

Lymphatic system - Structure and function

The lymphatic system consists of all lymphatic vessels and lymphoid organs. For example, the lymph nodes, spleen, thymus as well as the lymphatic tissue found in the small intestine (Peyer's patches) and throat (adenoid tonsils, palatine and tubal tonsils), to name a few, all represent lymphatic organs.

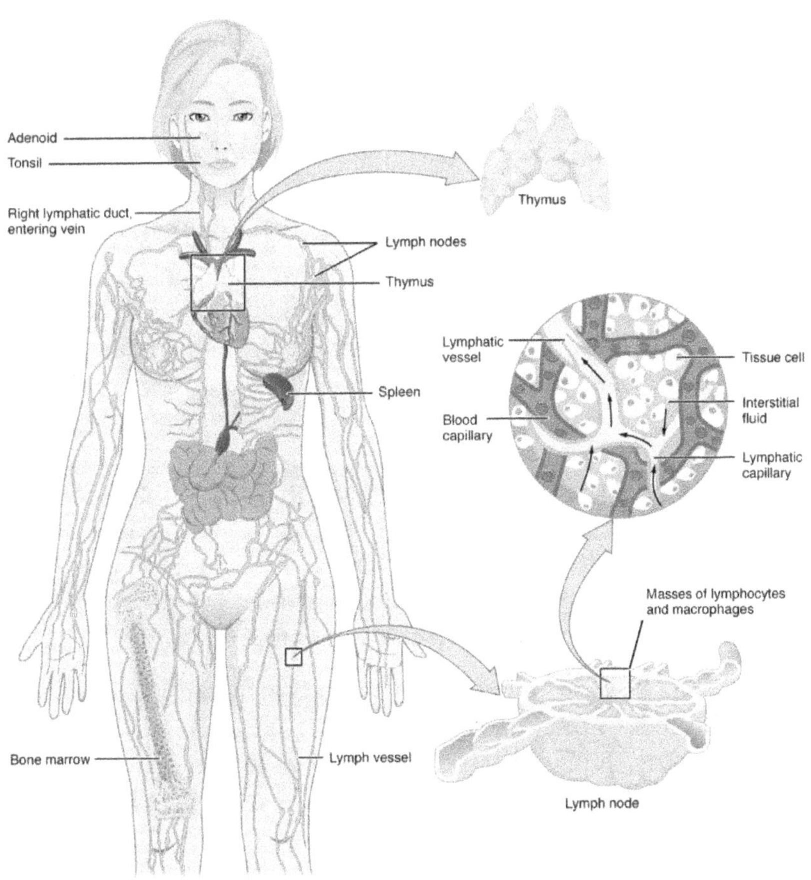

Hence, rather than representing a single organ, the lymphatic system comprises a circulatory network of vessels and lymphoid tissue and cells in every part of the body. It works together closely with the blood-producing (haematopoietic) system in the bone marrow, thereby playing a vital role in immune responses to protect the body from various pathogens. Also, the lymphatic vessel network helps transporting nutrients and waste products in the body.

Lymph and lymph vessels

The lymphatic system with its vessel network is – apart from the circulatory system, with which it is closely connected – the most important transport system in the human body.

The human body produces about two litres of lymph every day. This clear to yellow-tinted fluid is formed when blood plasma exits the capillary blood vessels and fills the small spaces (interstices) between and around body tissues and cells before being collected through small lymphatic vessels (lymph capillaries). The word lymph is derived from the name of the ancient Roman deity of fresh water, Lympha.

Lymph transports nutrients and oxygen for the cells as well as immune cells (such as lymphocytes). While circulating through the interstitial spaces of various tissues, lymph also picks up many of the body's waste products and carbon dioxide. Apart from that, lymph transports fat from the intestines to the blood.

After having been collected by the lymph capillaries, lymph is transported through larger lymphatic vessels to the lymph nodes, where lymphocytes purge it before it is emptied into the large (subclavian) veins close to the heart, where it blends again with the blood.

Lymph nodes

The network of lymphatic vessels includes multiple interposed lymph nodes, small lentil- or bean-sized organs. They serve as filter stations for the lymph of a certain body region and contain specials cells of the immune system, the lymphocytes, which fight infections attacking the body. Hence, the lymph nodes clean the lymph and free it from pathogens and infectious bodies.

The network of lymphatic vessels includes multiple interposed lymph nodes, small lentil- or bean-sized organs. They serve as filter stations for the lymph of a certain body region and contain specials cells of the immune system, the lymphocytes, which fight infections attacking the body. Hence, the lymph nodes clean the lymph and free it from pathogens and infectious bodies.

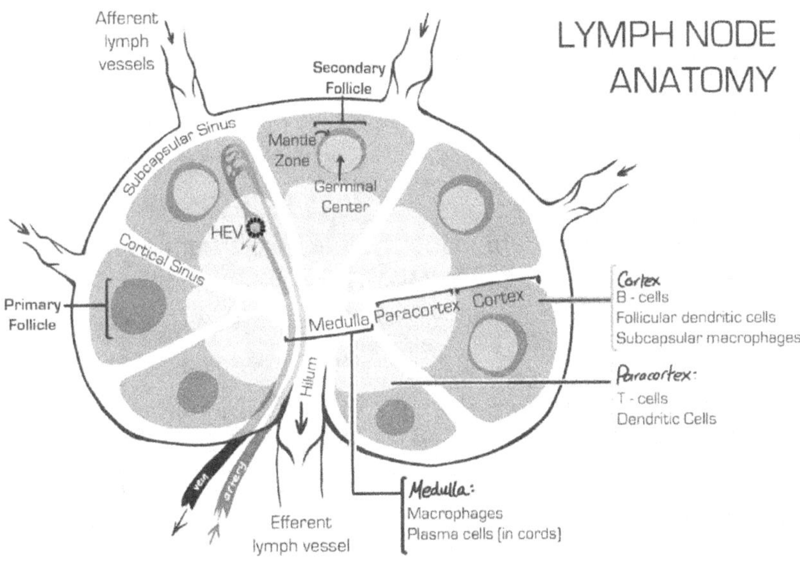

Spleen and thymus

The spleen is an organ in the left upper abdomen. Its job is to process old and damaged blood cells and microorganisms. Before birth, the spleen also helps producing blood cells. In early childhood, it plays a major role in building and maintaining the immune system.

The thymus is a gland located behind the breastbone (sternum). At birth, the thymus is the largest organ of the lymphatic system. It plays a vital role in building the immune system.

The thymus is also considered as the "school" of T-lymphocytes ("T" as in "Thymus"), because it teaches this subgroup of lymphocytes to differentiate between the body's own and alien immune cells. This means that in the thymus gland the T-lymphocytes learn and, thus, mature to be functional defence cells.

The organ keeps growing until puberty. In adults, it loses its size and relevance and its lymphatic tissue is mostly replaced by fat cells.

Lymphocytes

The cells of the lymphatic system, the lymphocytes, are a subgroup of the white blood cells. They play a major role within the body's immune defence, because they are able to target and eliminate pathogens.

Lymphocytes are formed like all other blood cells (such as all white and red blood cells as well as the platelets) – in the bone marrow, where they arise from blood precursor cells, the so-called blood stem cells (haematopoietic stem cells) and mature in a stepwise process.

The immediate precursor cells of lymphocytes are the so-called lymphoblasts. While passing several developmental stages both in the bone marrow and in various lymphatic organs (for example lymph nodes, spleen, thymus), they change their shape and features. When their development is completed, the mature, thus functioning lymphocytes are ready to leave the bone marrow or lymphatic organs, respectively, in order to fulfill their chores in blood and tissues.

The mature T- and B-lymphocytes subsequently reach the downstream lymphatic organs, such as spleen, lymph nodes, or tonsils. Both groups of lymphocytes serve the body's immune defence, however, with different functions.

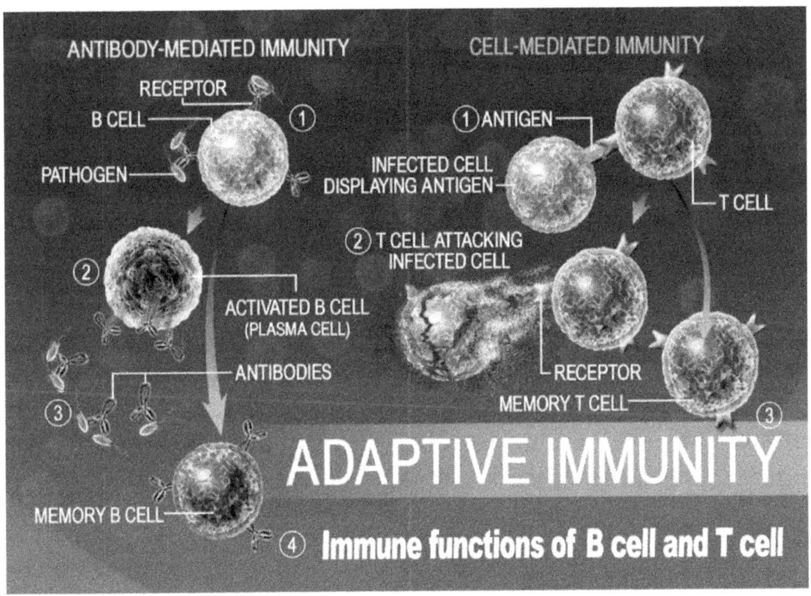

Depending on where their final maturation took place, lymphocytes are divided into two major groups: B-lymphocytes and T-lymphocytes. B-lymphocytes mature in the bone marrow, while the maturation of T-lymphocytes takes place in the thymus.

The mature T- and B-lymphocytes subsequently reach the downstream lymphatic organs, such as spleen, lymph nodes, or tonsils. Both groups of lymphocytes serve the body's immune defence, however, with different functions.

Functions of lymphocytes

A major task of mature B-lymphocytes, also known as plasma cells, is to produce antibodies. These are tiny protein molecules that stick to pathogens, thereby turning these into recognizable "enemies" to be engulfed, digested, or killed by so called "guzzle cells" (macrophages) or "natural killer cells" (special T-lymphocytes), respectively.

Natural killer cells are a subset of T-lymphocytes able to recognize and subsequently eliminate virus-infested cells as well as cancer cells. Other T-lymphocytes help the body to remember certain pathogens from

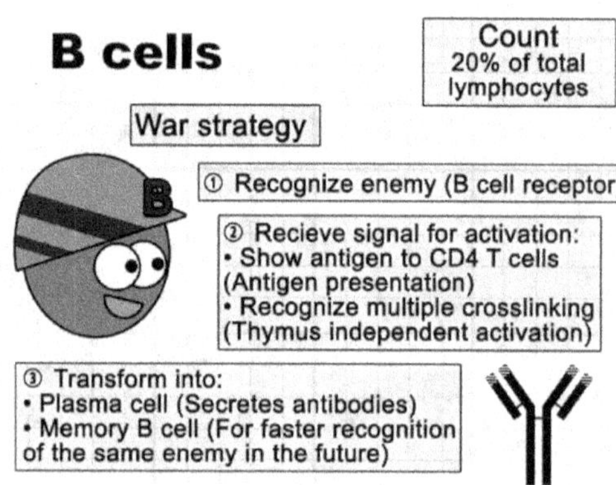

previous contacts. These "memory cells" basically organize the mission of the immune cells, thereby either activating or inhibiting the activity of the immune system.

The different subgroups of lymphocytes act in concert to fulfill their immunodefensive chores. They communicate via certain cellular messengers (hormones), the lymphokines. Taken together, the lymphatic system is a complex network of cells, tissues and regulatory mechanisms all working together to coordinate the body's immune system.

Lymphoma

Lymphoma is a type of cancer that affects the lymphatic system. The lymphatic system is a large network of vessels that carry a clear fluid, called lymph, that helps rid the body of germs, toxins, and other unwanted substances. Also included in the system are lymph nodes, the spleen, thymus gland, bone marrow, and a type of white blood cells known as lymphocytes. Lymphoma can affect any part of the lymphatic system and, in severe cases, spread to organs outside of the system.

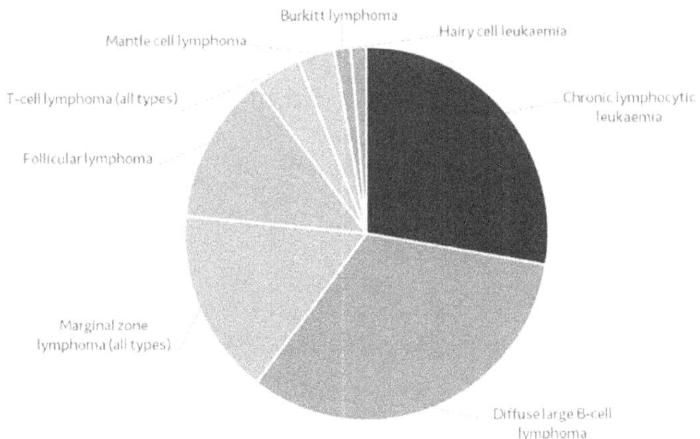

Types of Lymphoma

There are over 70 different types of lymphoma classified under the two broad categories:

Hodgkin lymphoma, marked by the presence of specific white blood cells called Reed-Sternberg cells, and generally more rare.

Non-Hodgkin lymphoma (NHL), marked by the absence of Reed-Sternberg cells, and generally more common.

NHL accounts for around 90% of all lymphomas and includes such subtypes as Burkitt lymphoma, chronic lymphocytic leukemia, diffuse large B-cell lymphoma, cutaneous B-cell lymphoma, cutaneous T-cell lymphoma, follicular lymphoma, and Waldenstrom macroglobulinemia.

The signs and symptoms of lymphoma are often nonspecific and may include swollen lymph nodes, fever, night sweats, and weight loss. If suspected, lymphoma can be definitively diagnosed with a lymph node biopsy, after which the disease will be categorized and staged to ensure the appropriate treatment.

According to the American Cancer Society, lymphoma is the fifth most common cancer in the United States—with over 82,000 new diagnoses each year—and the ninth leading cause of cancer deaths.

Non-Hodgkin lymphoma (NHL)

Non-Hodgkin lymphoma (NHL) is cancer that starts in lymphocytes, a type of white blood cell that helps fight infection. Lymphocytes are found in the blood stream but also in the lymph system and throughout the body. NHL most often affects adults and is more common than the other major category of lymphoma, Hodgkin lymphoma.

NHL refers to many different types of lymphoma that all share some characteristics. However, different types of NHL can behave very differently. The most common type is diffuse large B-cell lymphoma (DLBCL), an aggressive lymphoma. Other types may be more indolent, or slow-growing. Some can be cured, while others cannot. NHL treatments may include any number of agents such as chemotherapy, radiation, monoclonal antibodies, small molecules, cellular therapies or stem cell transplant.

Because lymphatic tissue is found in most parts of the body, NHL can start almost anywhere and can spread, or metastasize, to almost any organ. It often begins in the lymph nodes, liver, spleen, or bone marrow. However, it can also involve the stomach, intestines, skin, thyroid gland, brain, or any other part of the body.

Statistics

NHL is the seventh most common cancer in both men and women. The disease accounts for 4% of all cancers in the United States.

This year in 2020, an estimated 77,240 people (42,380 men and 34,860 women) in the United States will be diagnosed with NHL. While some subtypes of NHL are common in children, NHL is far more common in adults and risk increases with age. Over half of patients are age 65 or older when diagnosed. About 4,600 people ages 15 to 39 will be diagnosed with NHL this year.

It is estimated that 19,940 deaths (11,460 men and 8,480 women) from this disease will occur this year. It is the ninth most common cause of cancer death among both men and women. The survival rate has been improving since 1997, thanks to treatment advances. From 2008 to 2017, the death rate decreased by 2% annually.

The 5-year survival rate tells you what percent of people live at least 5 years after the cancer is found. Percent means how many out of 100. The overall 5-year survival rate for people with NHL is 72%.

For stage I NHL, the 5-year survival rate is more than 82%. For stage II the 5-year survival rate is 75% and for stage III it is 70%. For stage IV NHL, the 5-year survival rate is more than 62%. These survival rates vary depending on the cancer's stage and subtype.

It is important to remember that statistics on the survival rates for people with NHL are an estimate. The estimate comes from annual data based on the number of people with this cancer in the United States. Also, experts measure the survival statistics every 5 years. So the estimate may not show the results of better diagnosis or treatment available for less than 5 years. Talk with your doctor if you have any questions about this information.

Risk Factors of Lymphoma

Lymphoma is a group of blood cancers that develops when lymphocytes (a type of white blood cell) mutate and grow out of control. When this happens, the cancerous cells no longer die but continue to multiply and invade different parts of the body. Although genetics plays a central role in the development of lymphoma, no one knows for sure what causes the cells to mutate.

What scientists do know is that certain risk factors can increase your risk of lymphoma. Having one or more of these risk factors does not mean you will get lymphoma. In most cases, they can't even predict your likelihood of developing the disease. Still, they may provide your doctor with valuable clues that can lead to an early diagnosis and treatment.

The key risk factors associated with lymphoma include:

- Age
- Sex
- Immune dysfunction
- Family history
- Certain infections
- Chemical exposure
- Previous cancers and cancer treatments
- Obesity and diet may also play a part.

Common Risk Factors

Lymphoma is not a single disease but a group of related blood cancers with numerous types and subtypes. The two main types are Hodgkin lymphoma and non-Hodgkin lymphoma. Both of these lymphomas differ not only in their disease pattern and cell types but also in many of their risk factors.

Many of these risk factors are non-modifiable, meaning that there is nothing you can do to change them. Chief among them are age, sex, and immune dysfunction.

Age

Age plays a key role in the development of lymphoma. Although lymphoma can occur at any age, including childhood, the majority are diagnosed in adults over 60.

However, unlike non-Hodgkin lymphoma, a significant number of Hodgkin lymphoma cases are diagnosed between the ages of 15 and 40. Because of this, the median age for diagnosis of non-Hodgkin lymphoma is 55, whereas the median age for diagnosis of Hodgkin lymphoma is 39.

Sex

Sex is another risk factor that places some individuals at greater risk of lymphoma than others. While men are slightly more likely to develop lymphoma than women, there are certain types of lymphoma for which women are at greater risk. This includes nodular sclerosing Hodgkin's lymphoma (the most common and treatable form of Hodgkin lymphoma) as well as non-Hodgkin lymphoma of the breast, thyroid, and the respiratory tract.

It is believed that the hormone estrogen influences which types of lymphoma are more or less common in women. There are also variations in how women respond to certain therapies, with women generally responding better to drugs like Rituxan (rituximab) and Revlimid (lenalidomide) than men. □

Immune Dysfunction

The immune system plays a central role in the development of lymphoma, in part by suppressing mutations in the two main types of lymphocytes (called B-cells and T-cells) that can lead to cancer.

As you get older, your immune response will invariably begin to weaken. This may explain why lymphoma is more common in people over 60 and why the risk continues to grow every year thereafter. But, age is not the only factor that contributes to the loss of immune function.

Advanced HIV infection, characterized by the severe depletion of T-cells, is known to increase the risk of a rare form of lymphoma known as lymphocyte-depleted Hodgkin lymphoma (LHDL).

A similar situation is seen with organ transplant recipients who need immunosuppressant drugs to prevent organ rejection. In this group of people, there is a high risk of non-Hodgkin lymphomas, most especially hepatosplenic T-cell lymphoma, Burkitt lymphoma, and diffuse large B-cell lymphoma.

Certain autoimmune diseases are also linked to increased rates of lymphoma, although it is not entirely clear why. According to a 2008 study published in the journal Blood, people with lupus and Sjögren syndrome have as much as a seven-fold increased risk of non-Hodgkin lymphoma compared to the general population.

Genetics

Another risk factor you can't change are your genetics. Although there is no single gene that "causes" lymphoma, there are some that may predispose you to the disease. In recent years, scientists have begun to link specific genetic mutations to specific types of lymphoma.

These include mutations involving oncogenes, which help cells grow and divide, and tumor suppressor genes, which tell a cell when it is time to die. If either (or both) of these genes mutate, cells can suddenly multiply and spread out of control without end. Many scientists believe that a combination of mutations is needed to induce lymphoma (a hypothesis referred to as the "multi-hit theory") □

This is evidenced in part by the pattern of inheritance in families. Unlike autosomal dominant disorders in which there is a 50/50 chance of developing a disease if a gene is inherited, lymphoma doesn't have a clear pattern of inheritance. Still, family history plays a central role in the overall risk, most specifically with Hodgkin lymphoma.

Research published in a 2015 edition of Blood concluded that having a first-degree relative (parent or sibling) with Hodgkin lymphoma increases your risk of the disease by 3-fold compared to the general population.

The inheritance pattern in families with non-Hodgkin lymphoma is far less clear. Although there is a modest familial risk, the current body of evidence suggests that the genetic mutations are more often acquired than inherited. This may be caused by exposure to radiation, chemicals, or infections or occur spontaneously with advancing age or for no apparent reason at all. □

Infectious and Environmental Causes

A number of infections, environmental toxins, and medical treatments have been linked to lymphoma. Scientists believe that they either trigger the disease in people genetically predisposed to lymphoma or cause the mutations themselves.

Infections

A number of bacterial, viral, and parasitic infections are known to increase the risk of lymphoma. Among them:

Campylobacter jejuni is a common cause of bacterial food poisoning that is linked to a type of abdominal lymphoma known as immunoproliferative small intestinal disease.

Cellulitis, a severe bacterial skin infection, is with a 15% to 28% increased risk of non-Hodgkin lymphoma, most especially cutaneous T-cell lymphoma. □

Chlamydophila psittaci, a bacteria associated with the lung infection psittacosis, is linked to ocular adnexal marginal zone lymphoma (lymphoma of the eye).

Epstein-Barr virus (EBV) is closely linked to both Burkitt lymphoma and post-transplant lymphoma, as well as 20% to 25% of all Hodgkin lymphoma cases.

Helicobacter pylori (H. pylori), a bacterial infection associated with gastric ulcers, is linked to mucosa-associated lymphoid tissue (MALT) lymphoma of the stomach.

Hepatitis C virus (HCV) can increase the risk of non-Hodgkin lymphoma by causing the excessive production of lymphocytes, many of which are malformed and vulnerable to malignancy. Lymphomas linked to HCV are generally low-grade and slow-growing.

Human herpesvirus 8 (HHV8), a virus associated with a rare skin cancer called Kaposi sarcoma in people with HIV, can increase the risk of an equally rare lymphoma known as primary effusion lymphoma (PEL).

Human T-cell lymphotropic virus (HTLV-1), a virus spread by blood transfusions, sexual contact, and shared needles, is closely linked to highly aggressive adult T-cell leukemia/lymphoma (ATL).

Environmental Toxins

Some studies have suggested that chemicals like benzene and certain insecticides are linked with an increased risk of both Hodgkin and non-Hodgkin lymphoma. It is a highly contentious topic, with some studies suggesting an increased risk of lymphoma and others showing no risk at all.

A 2013 study published in Cancer Causes and Control found a close association between Hodgkin lymphoma and the use of insecticides and fungicides (especially those containing acetylcholinesterase inhibitors found in products like Baygon). Interestingly, the risk was limited to adults who used five or more insecticides, making it less clear which substances pose the greatest harm.

A Canadian study published in the International Journal of Cancer similarly found that people with non-Hodgkin lymphoma had higher levels of pesticide chemicals in their blood than people without. Chief among these were pesticides containing chlordane (a chemical banned in the United States since 1988), which reportedly increased the risk of non-Hodgkin lymphoma by 2.7 fold.

Further research is needed to determine how these chemical toxins contribute to lymphoma and what risk they actually pose.

Cancer Therapy

Both chemotherapy and radiation therapy used to treat cancer can increase a person's risk of lymphoma. With that said, the risk has been decreasing in recent years due to newer drugs and safer radiotherapy techniques.

The risk of lymphoma is seen to increase with the aggressiveness of the therapy. For example, BEACOPP chemotherapy, involving seven different drugs, is more likely to cause second cancers than CHOP regimens involving four. The duration of therapy and the incidence of relapse also play a part.

According to a 2011 study in Annals of Oncology. the use of BEACOPP in people with relapsed lymphoma increases the likelihood of a second relapse by 660%.

BEACOPP also increases the risk of acute myeloid leukemia (AML) and myelodysplastic syndrome (MDS) by 450%.

People previously exposed to high levels of radiation therapy are also at an increased risk of lymphoma. The risk is especially high in people with non-small cell lung cancer in whom radiation can increase the risk of non-Hodgkin lymphoma by as much as 53%. The risk is further increased when radiation and chemotherapy are combined.

To reduce the risk, radiology oncologists have largely replaced extended field radiation (EFR) with involved-field radiation therapy (IFRT) which employs a narrower, more focused beam of radiation.

Lifestyle Factors

Certain lifestyle factors can increase your risk of lymphoma. Although there are things you can do to modify these factors, it is not entirely clear how much the changes will impact your risk.

Obesity

A number of studies have found a direct link between obesity and Hodgkin lymphoma, with an increasing body mass index (BMI) corresponding to an increased risk of lymphoma.

According to a 2019 study in the British Journal of Cancer, every 5 kg/m^2 increase in BMI is associated with a 10% increase in the risk of Hodgkin lymphoma.

The study, which looked at the impact of obesity in 5.8 million people in the United Kingdom, concluded that 7.4% percent of adult lymphoma cases can be attributed to being overweight (BMI over 25) or obese (BMI over 30).

Despite early claims that certain fats are linked to gastrointestinal lymphoma, most scientists agree that the type of fat consumed is less important than the impact of body weight on lymphoma. With that said, trans fats are linked to a significantly higher incidence of non-Hodgkin lymphoma in women.

Whether losing weight will reduce the risk of lymphoma on an individual basis is unclear. Even so, maintaining a healthy diet and an ideal weight is beneficial to your health and can help support immune function.

Breast Implants

Another less common risk factor involves breast implants. Although rare, some women with implants have been known to develop anaplastic large cell lymphoma (ALCL) in their breast. This seems more likely with implants that are textured rather than those that are smooth. While selecting a smooth implant can theoretically reduce your risk, the overall risk irrespective of implant type is only around one per 1,000 procedures.

Types of NHL

First, the doctor will determine what type of cell the lymphoma started in and classify the disease within 1 of the 3 major groups:

B-cell lymphoma - About 90% of people in western countries with lymphoma have B-cell lymphoma.

T-cell lymphoma - About 10% of people with lymphoma have T-cell lymphoma. These lymphomas are more frequent in Asian countries.

NK-cell lymphoma - Less than 1% of people with lymphoma have NK-cell lymphoma.

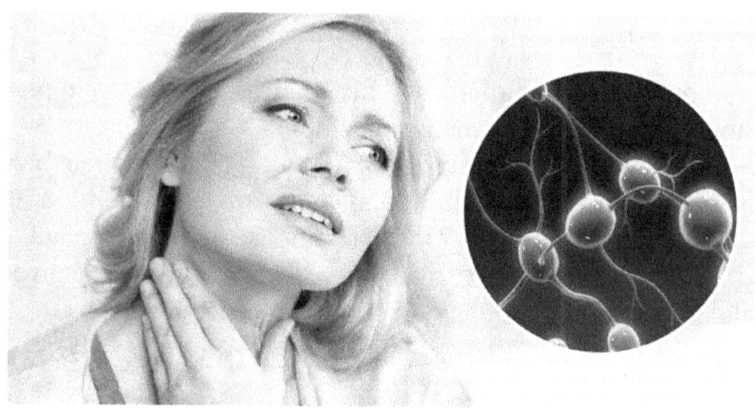

NHL is also described by how quickly the cancer is growing, either "indolent" or "aggressive." Indolent and aggressive NHL are equally common in adults. In children, aggressive NHL is more common. Some subtypes of lymphoma cannot easily be classified as indolent or aggressive. For example, mantle cell lymphoma has both indolent and aggressive NHL features.

Indolent NHL

These types of lymphoma grow slowly. As a result, people with indolent NHL may not need to start treatment when it is first diagnosed. They are followed closely, and treatment is only usually started when they develop symptoms or the disease begins to change. This is called watchful waiting or active surveillance. In cases where there are many cancer cells in the body, called high-burden disease, treatment will be started even if there are no symptoms.

When indolent lymphoma is located only in 1 or 2 adjacent areas, it is called localized disease (stages I and II). For people with localized disease, radiation therapy is often used. However, most patients with indolent NHL have stage III or IV disease at the time of diagnosis. There are many effective treatments for these stages of indolent NHL. However, it may come back months or years after treatment has finished and require more treatment.

Aggressive NHL

These types of lymphoma may develop rapidly, and treatment is usually started within weeks. These types of lymphoma usually need more intensive chemotherapy. The doctor may recommend adding radiation therapy to treat stage I or II disease or to treat lymphoma where the site of the disease is large, sometimes called "bulky" disease. Some forms of aggressive lymphoma may be cured with effective treatment.

Subtypes of NHL

In addition to determining if the NHL is indolent or aggressive and whether it is B-cell, T-cell, or NK-cell lymphoma, it is very important to determine the subtype of NHL. This is because each subtype can behave differently and may require different treatments. There are more than 60 NHL subtypes, although some are quite rare.

There are more than 60 types of lymphoma

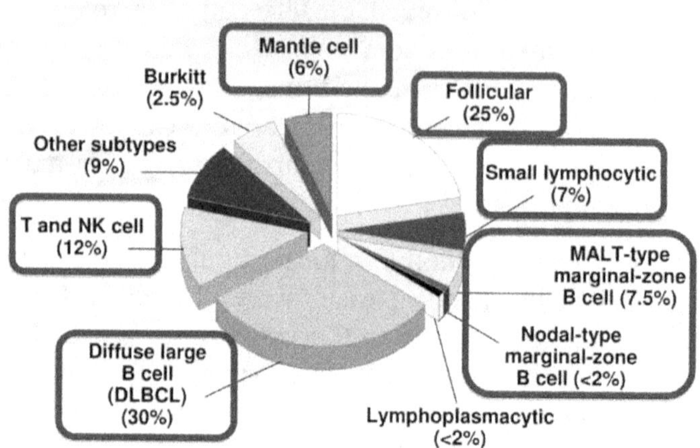

Distinguishing among the different subtypes of NHL can be difficult and requires pathologists or hematopathologists who are experts in the diagnosis of lymphoma. These specialists use sophisticated techniques and work closely with experienced oncologists. The diagnosis is based on how the lymphoma looks under the microscope. The doctors confirm the diagnosis with additional information from other tests, including tests of genetic material within the lymphoma cells.

Subtypes of B-cell lymphoma

These are the common subtypes of B-cell lymphoma.

Diffuse large B-cell lymphoma (DLBCL)

DLBCL is the most common form of lymphoma. About 30% of NHL in the United States is DLBCL. It is an aggressive form of NHL that involves organs other than the lymph nodes about 40% of the time. About 2 out of 3 people with DLBCL are cured with chemotherapy given in combination with rituximab (Rituxan). Radiation therapy is also used for some people, especially if the lymphoma is found in a limited area. Your doctor may check the fluid around the brain, called cerebrospinal fluid (CSF), in certain cases at diagnosis and recommend treatments to prevent the lymphoma from spreading to the brain, called central nervous system (CNS) prophylaxis. However, most people do not need this type of treatment.

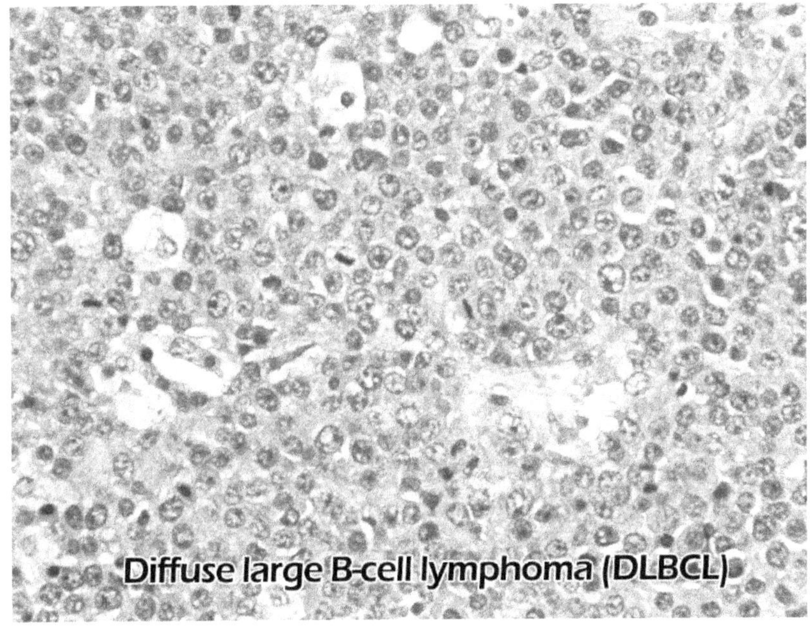

Follicular lymphoma

Follicular lymphoma is the second most common form of lymphoma in the United States and Europe. About 20% of people with NHL have this subtype. It usually begins in the lymph nodes, is most often indolent, and grows very slowly. People with early, stage I follicular lymphoma may be cured with radiation therapy. For some, bone marrow/stem cell transplantation may cure the disease. Patients with follicular lymphoma may receive a combination of chemotherapy, targeted therapy, and/or radiation therapy. Or, they may be followed closely with watchful waiting and start treatment only when symptoms appear.

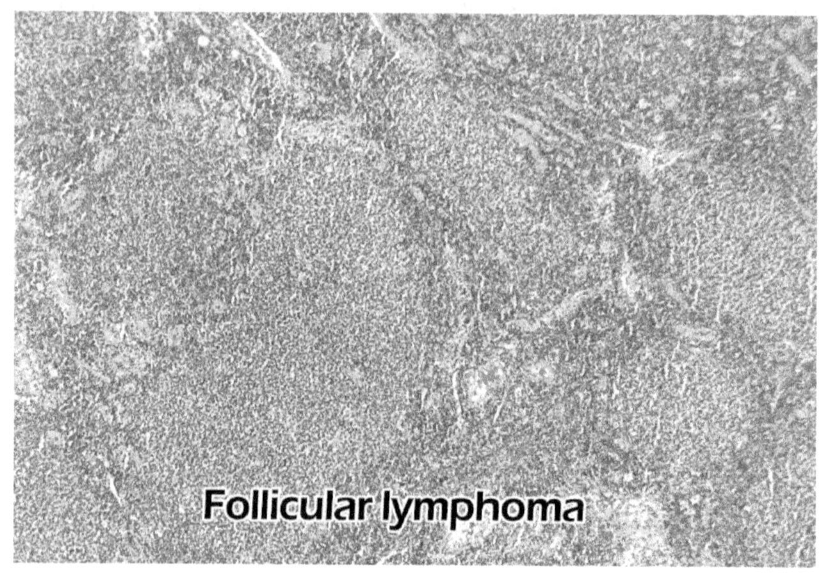

Recent clinical trials suggest that people with follicular lymphoma have lived longer over the last few decades. Research shows that some monoclonal antibodies alone or in combination with drugs such as bendamustine (Treanda) and lenalidomide (Revlimid) are effective for this subtype. There are many new drugs being tested for the treatment of follicular lymphoma. Over time, follicular lymphoma may turn into DLBCL (see above), which will then require more aggressive treatment. This is called transformation. If follicular lymphoma transforms, it can be treated the same way as DLBCL.

Localized radiation therapy is often a common treatment choice for people with stage I follicular lymphoma and for some people with stage II follicular lymphoma.

Mantle cell lymphoma

About 5% to 7% of people with NHL have mantle cell lymphoma. It most often appears in people older than 60 and is much more common in men than in women. It usually involves the bone marrow, lymph nodes, spleen, and gastrointestinal system, which includes the esophagus, stomach, and intestines. Mantle cell lymphoma is identified by a protein called cyclin D1 or by a genetic change within the lymphoma cells involving chromosomes 11 and 14. Some patients have a slower-growing form of the disease and if they do not have symptoms or a significant amount of disease, some may be monitored using the watchful waiting approach.

Treatment of mantle cell lymphoma often uses a combination of chemotherapy and a monoclonal antibody, which is a type of targeted therapy. For younger patients who are otherwise healthy, high-dose chemotherapy and autologous bone marrow transplantation often results in the longest remission, and they may receive maintenance therapy with the rituximab. For older patients or those who are not able to receive an autologous bone marrow transplant, maintenance therapy with rituximab is a standard treatment approach.

If chemotherapy does not work or the disease comes back, called recurrence, there are differing opinions on the best way to treat mantle cell lymphoma. Research shows that drugs such as acalabrutinib (Calquence), ibrutinib (Imbruvica), and lenalidomide may be effective. Researchers are studying these drugs as part of first-line treatment. Researchers are also studying new drugs for mantle cell lymphoma.

Small lymphocytic lymphoma

This type of lymphoma is the same disease as B-cell chronic lymphocytic leukemia (CLL) without a significant amount of disease in the blood. About 5% of people with NHL have this subtype, which is considered indolent lymphoma. People with small lymphocytic lymphoma may not require treatment, but instead receive watchful waiting. Some patients receive a combination of chemotherapy and a targeted therapy.

First-line treatment may include a combination of ibrutinib and obinutuzumab (Gazyva), which is a monoclonal antibody. Ibrutinib alone is also approved by the U.S. Food and Drug Administration (FDA) to treat small lymphocytic lymphoma that has come back after treatment. Another targeted therapy, venetoclax (Venclexta), in combination with obinutuzumab is approved as a first treatment for small lymphocytic lymphoma. Venetoclax may also be used in combination with rituximab.

Double hit/triple hit lymphoma

This is a highly aggressive subtype, accounting for about 5% of cases. Rarely, low-grade follicular lymphoma may also transform into double hit lymphoma. Double hit lymphomas have changes in the MYC gene and in either the BCL2 or BCL6 gene. Double hit lymphoma is often diagnosed in older adults. There is currently no established treatment regimen, although combinations of chemotherapy and rituximab are the most common options. Triple hit lymphomas have changes in the MYC, BCL2, and BCL6 genes.

Primary mediastinal large B-cell lymphoma

This is an aggressive form of DLBCL. It appears as a large mass in the chest area. The mass may cause breathing problems or superior vena cava (SVC) syndrome, a collection of symptoms caused by the partial blockage or compression of the superior vena cava. The superior vena cava is the major vein that carries blood from the head, neck, upper chest, and arms to the heart. Mediastinal large B-cell lymphoma is most common in women between 30 and 40 years old. About 2.5% of people with NHL have this subtype. Most often, doctors treat it with combination chemotherapy plus rituximab. Radiation therapy to the chest may be used in people for whom chemotherapy did not work. For lymphoma that has not responded to chemotherapy and radiation, CAR T-cell therapy may be an option. A closely related lymphoma called mediastinal grey-zone lymphoma (MGZL) may also occur in the same age group. It is treated in a manner similar to that of primary mediastinal large B-cell lymphoma.

Splenic marginal zone B-cell lymphoma

This type of lymphoma begins in the spleen and usually involves the bone marrow and the blood. It is usually slow growing, and the treatment approach is often watchful waiting. If treatment is needed, rituximab is often used, although some patients may also need chemotherapy. In some circumstances, surgical removal of the spleen may be needed.

Extranodal marginal zone B-cell lymphoma MALT

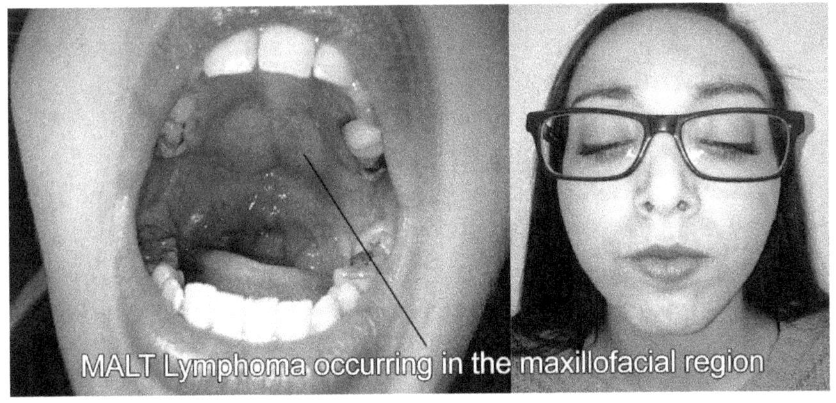

This type of lymphoma most commonly occurs in the stomach. However, it may also occur in the lung, skin, thyroid, salivary gland, or in the orbit, adjacent to the eye, or in the bowel. Patients with this type of lymphoma sometimes have a history of autoimmune disease, such as lupus, rheumatoid arthritis, or Sjögren syndrome. When MALT occurs in the stomach, it is sometimes caused by a bacteria called Helicobacter pylori. When MALT is caused by this bacteria, antibiotics can sometimes effectively treat the disease. For disease only affecting only 1 organ, radiation therapy can sometimes cure MALT. Rituximab with or without chemotherapy is also sometimes used to treat MALT.

Nodal marginal zone B-cell lymphoma

This rare type of indolent lymphoma involves the lymph nodes. About 1% of people with lymphoma have this subtype. In general, doctors treat this subtype of lymphoma similarly to follicular lymphoma.

Lymphoplasmacytic lymphoma

This is an indolent form of lymphoma, and 1% of people with NHL have this subtype. This form of lymphoma often involves the bone marrow, sometimes lymph nodes, and spleen. In many patients, this lymphoma produces a protein, called an "M protein," that is found in the blood. When this occurs, the condition is called Waldenstrom's macroglobulinemia (WM). Patients with WM sometimes have elevated serum viscosity, or "thickened" blood, which may cause symptoms such as headache, blurry vision, dizziness, and shortness of breath. Changes in the MYD88 gene are detected in more than 90% of cases of lymphoplasmacytic lymphoma and WM. Looking for mutations in this gene may be helpful in diagnosing lymphoplasmacytic lymphoma. Treatment may include:

- Watchful waiting
- Chemotherapy
- Targeted therapy with monoclonal antibodies
- Combinations of chemotherapy and monoclonal antibodies

Clinical trial researchers are studying using chemotherapy followed by bone marrow transplantation as a treatment option, which may be useful if the lymphoma returns after initial treatment.

Primary effusion lymphoma

This rare and very aggressive form of lymphoma most often occurs in people:

- Who have the human immunodeficiency virus (HIV), which causes autoimmune deficiency syndrome (AIDS)
- Whose immune system does not work well for other reasons
- Who are elderly

This lymphoma often shows up as fluid around the lung, heart, or abdominal cavity. Often, there are no tumor masses. It is treated the same way as other diffuse large-cell lymphomas.

Burkitt lymphoma

This is a very rare and aggressive form of lymphoma. There are 3 forms of Burkitt ymphoma:

- Endemic
- Sporadic
- Immunodeficiency-related lymphoma

The endemic subtype occurs most commonly in Africa, appears most often in the jawbones of children, and is usually associated with infection with EBV. It can also be associated with HIV. In the United States, Burkitt lymphoma sometimes

appears with a mass in the abdomen, but it can affect many other parts of the body. Because this type of lymphoma spreads quickly, it

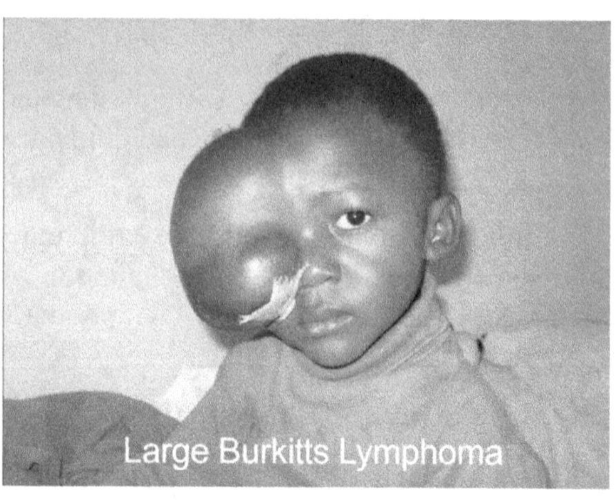

needs immediate treatment. This subtype often has abnormalities involving the MYC gene, which can contribute to cancer growth.

Burkitt lymphoma is often curable. A series of treatments with chemotherapy, each usually given over several days in a hospital, can lead to long-term remission in more than 80% of patients.

Subtypes of T-cell and NK-cell lymphoma

These are the most common subtypes of T-cell and NK-cell lymphoma:

Anaplastic large cell lymphoma, primary cutaneous

This subtype of lymphoma only involves the skin. It is often indolent, although aggressive subtypes of the disease are possible. When the cancer is localized, radiation therapy is often effective. If it has spread, chemotherapy is the usual treatment. New drugs have recently been developed for the treatment of cutaneous lymphomas.

Anaplastic large cell lymphoma, systemic

This form makes up about 2% of all lymphomas and about 10% of all childhood lymphomas. In people with this subtype, an increased amount of the ALK-1 protein may be found in the cancer cells. Those who have ALK-1 protein in the cancer cells often have a better prognosis than those who do not have the ALK-1 protein in the cancer cells. This is an aggressive form of lymphoma, but chemotherapy often works well. New treatments, such as the targeted therapy brentuximab vedotin (Adcetris) or bone marrow transplantation, may sometimes be a treatment option.

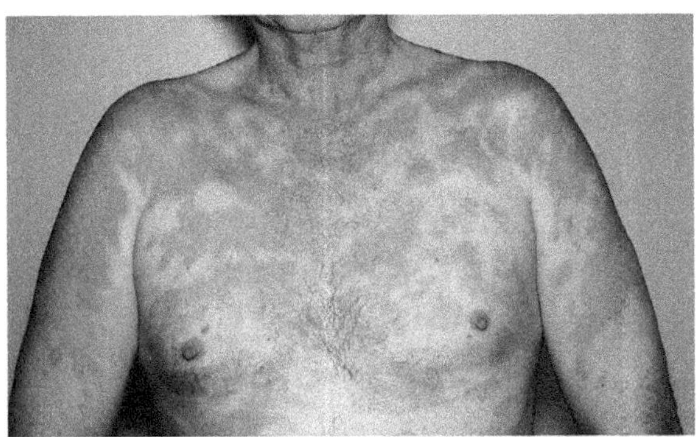

Breast implant-associated anaplastic large cell lymphoma

This is a relatively recently recognized subtype that arises in areas near breast implants. It is usually less aggressive than the systemic type of anaplastic large cell lymphoma, and treatment includes surgical removal of the implant.

Peripheral T-cell lymphoma, not otherwise specified (NOS)

This is an aggressive form of lymphoma that is often advanced when doctors find it. It is most common in people older than 60 and makes up about 6% of all lymphomas in the United

States and Europe. The cells of this lymphoma vary in size, and they have certain types of proteins, called CD4 or CD8, on their surface. It is treated with chemotherapy. Researchers are studying many new drugs in clinical trials to treat this subtype. Bone marrow transplantation may sometimes be an option.

Angioimmunoblastic T-cell lymphoma

This is an aggressive form of lymphoma with specific symptoms:

- Enlarged, often tender, lymph nodes
- Fever
- Weight loss
- Rash
- High levels of immunoglobulins in the blood

Patients with angioimmunoblastic lymphoma have lowered immune system functions, so infections are also common. Doctors identify this type of lymphoma by what it looks like under a microscope and by certain proteins found in the tumor cells. It is treated like other aggressive lymphomas.

Adult T-cell lymphoma/leukemia (human T-cell lymphotropic virus type I positive)

This type of lymphoma is caused by a virus called the human T-cell lymphotropic virus type I. It is an aggressive disease that often involves the bone and skin. Often, lymphoma cells are found in the blood, which is why this condition is sometimes also called leukemia. Chemotherapy does not usually work well for this form of lymphoma, although interferon and zidovudine (Retrovir) help some patients. Allogenic (ALLO) bone marrow transplantation may be the best approach for treatment of this type of lymphoma in people whose disease is under control after chemotherapy.

Extranodal NK/T-cell lymphoma, nasal type

This is an aggressive type of lymphoma that is very rare in the United States and Europe in general, but more common in Asian and Hispanic communities. It can occur in children or adults, most often involving the nasal area and sinuses. It can also involve the gastrointestinal tract, skin, the testicles, or other areas in the body. Radiation therapy in combination with chemotherapy is an important part of the treatment for disease that involves the nasal/sinus area. This subtype responds well to chemotherapy with asparaginase (Elspar), and some people may benefit from a bone marrow transplant.

Enteropathy-associated T-cell lymphoma

This type of lymphoma is rare in the United States but is more common in Europe. It is an aggressive form of T-cell lymphoma that involves the intestines. Some people with this subtype have celiac disease or a history of gluten intolerance. High-dose chemotherapy may be used to treat the disease.

Hepatosplenic T-cell lymphoma

This is an aggressive form of peripheral T-cell lymphoma that involves the liver and spleen. The disease occurs most often in teenaged and young men. It is usually managed with chemotherapy followed by ALLO bone marrow transplantation.

Subcutaneous panniculitis-like T-cell lymphoma

This is a form of peripheral T-cell lymphoma that is similar to hepatosplenic T-cell lymphoma. The disease involves the tissue under the skin and is often first diagnosed as panniculitis, which is inflammation of fatty tissues. It is treated as a high-risk aggressive lymphoma.

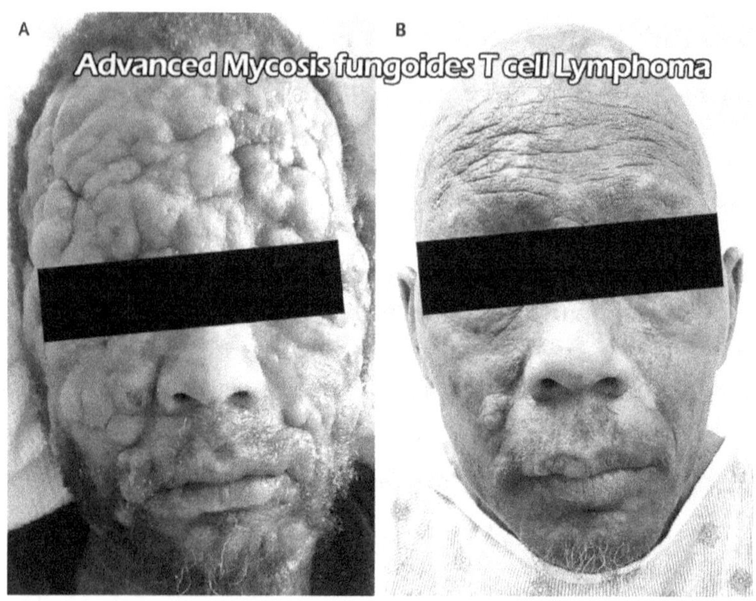

Mycosis fungoides

This is a rare T-cell lymphoma that primarily involves the skin. It often has a very long and indolent course but may become more aggressive and spread to lymph nodes or internal organs. Mycosis fungoides can be managed with topical medications, controlled exposure to specialized radiation in the form of lights or radiation therapy, and systemic treatments, such as chemotherapy or targeted therapy. This type of NHL usually cannot be cured, but it is often manageable.

Symptoms, and Complications

The distinction between HL and NHL is made by looking at a sample of biopsied tissue under the microscope. With HL, there will be abnormal cells with two nuclei, called Reed-Sternberg cells, that do not occur with NHL.

Despite the cellular differences, both HL and NHL have many of the same symptoms, particularly in the early stages of the disease.

However, the pathogenesis (the manner in which the disease develops) differs significantly from one lymphoma subtype to the next. Some lymphomas develop in an orderly fashion as this malignancy moves through the lymphatic system (comprised of the lymph nodes, spleen, tonsils, thymus gland, and bone marrow).

Others develop haphazardly, establishing tumors in specific parts of the lymphatic system or moving outside of the system to affect distant organs.

The warning signs of lymphoma can often be so subtle that it may take years before you realize that anything is wrong. Moreover, many of the symptoms will be non-specific and easily confused with other, less serious diseases. Even so, there are tell-tale clues to watch out for if you think you may have lymphoma or have a family history of the disease.

Frequent Symptoms

The lymphatic system is a closed network of vessels and organs whose role is it to isolate and kill germs in the body. Central to this system are lymphocytes and lymph nodes.

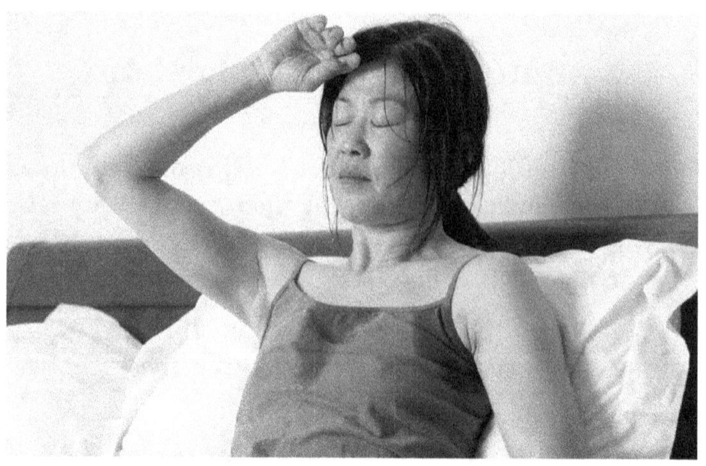

Like all white blood cells, lymphocytes are part of the body's first line of defense against infection. They are transported throughout the vascular network of the lymphatic system in a fluid known as lymph. Scattered along the route are dense clusters of lymph nodes whose role it is to filter bacteria, viruses, and other microorganisms from lymph.

Under normal circumstances, lymphocytes move in and out of the lymph nodes freely to carry on their immune functions. When lymphoma develops, they will start to accumulate in the lymph nodes in an attempt to isolate and neutralize the malignancy.

This accumulation, along with the destruction of other white blood cells known as macrophages and monocytes, can lead to a cascade of symptoms characteristic to both HL and NHL, including:

- Lymphadenopathy (swollen lymph nodes)
- Fever
- Night sweats
- Anorexia (loss of appetite)
- Pruritus (itching)

- Dyspnea (shortness of breath)
- Unintended weight loss
- Persistent fatigue

Lymphadenopathy Types

Of all of the symptoms, lymphadenopathy is the central defining feature. The swollen nodes will typically be described as being firm, rubbery, and movable in the surrounding tissues. Unlike the tender lymph nodes associated with viral infections like HIV, lymphadenopathy caused by lymphoma is rarely painful.

For reasons unknown, lymph node pain can occur immediately after drinking alcohol, providing what may be the warning sign of lymphoma.

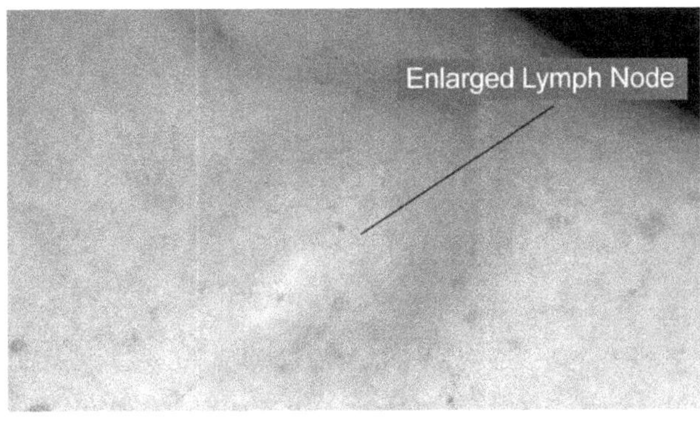

The location of lymphadenopathy can also provide clues as to the type of lymphoma involved:

With HL, which moves in a sequential fashion through the lymphatic system, lymphadenopathy will almost invariably start in the upper body—typically the neck (cervical lymph nodes), chest (mediastinal lymph nodes), or armpits (axillary lymph nodes)—before progressing to the lower body.

With NHL, the disease develops haphazardly and can affect lymph nodes in any part of the body, including the abdomen (peritoneal lymph nodes) and groin (inguinal lymph nodes).

The very fact that you have swollen lymph nodes that do not resolve should be the first clue that you need to see a doctor.

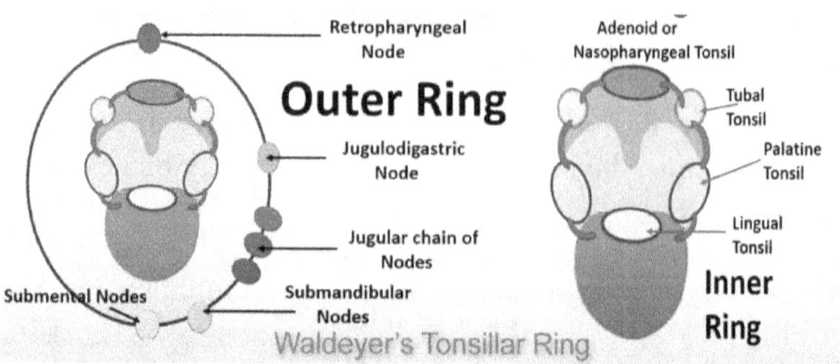

Extranodal Symptoms

The symptoms of lymphoma are defined by the type and subtype of lymphoma involved as well as its stage, and grade (severity), and location in the body. This is especially true if the disease is extranodal, meaning that it occurs outside of the lymph nodes.

There are two main categories of extranodal lymphoma:

Primary extranodal lymphoma occurs when the disease originates outside of the lymphatic system. The vast majority of primary extranodal cases occur with NHL; it is exceptionally rare with HL.

Secondary extranodal lymphoma originates in the lymphatic system and then spreads to other organs. This can occur with both HL and NHL.

The definition of extranodal can vary slightly based on whether HL or NHL is involved. With HL, the spleen, tonsils, and thymus are considered nodal sites since the disease spreads within the confines of the lymphatic system. By contrast, these same organs are considered extranodal with NHL given that the disease develops spontaneously in any part of the body.

While nodal lymphoma is characterized by lymphadenopathy and other classic symptoms, the symptoms of extranodal lymphoma are dictated by the organs affected.

Gastrointestinal Tract

The stomach and small intestine are the first and second most common sites for extranodal lymphoma. Primary NHL is the usual culprit, with most stomach lymphomas linked to a type known as mucosa-associated lymphoid tissue (MALT) lymphoma. The types of NHL affecting the small intestine include MALT, mantle cell lymphoma, Burkitt lymphoma, and enteropathy-associated lymphoma.

Symptoms of gastrointestinal lymphoma may include:

- Abdominal tenderness and pain
- Cramps
- Indigestion
- Constipation
- Diarrhea
- Malaise (a general feeling of unwellness)
- Early satiation (a feeling of fullness after a few bites)
- Nausea and vomiting
- Rectal bleeding
- Black, tarry stools
- Unintended weight loss ☐
- Skin

Cutaneous (skin) lymphoma

occurs with both HL and NHL. Around 25% of nodal lymphomas will manifest with skin symptoms, while 65% of all NHL cases will be attributed to a subtype known as cutaneous T-cell lymphoma. One of the most common subtypes is mycosis fungoides.

Symptoms of cutaneous lymphoma may include:

- Round skin patches that may be raised, scaly, or itchy
- Lightened patches of skin
- Skin tumors that can spontaneously break open
- Thickening of the palms or soles
- An itchy, rash-like redness covering much of the body
- Alopecia (hair loss)

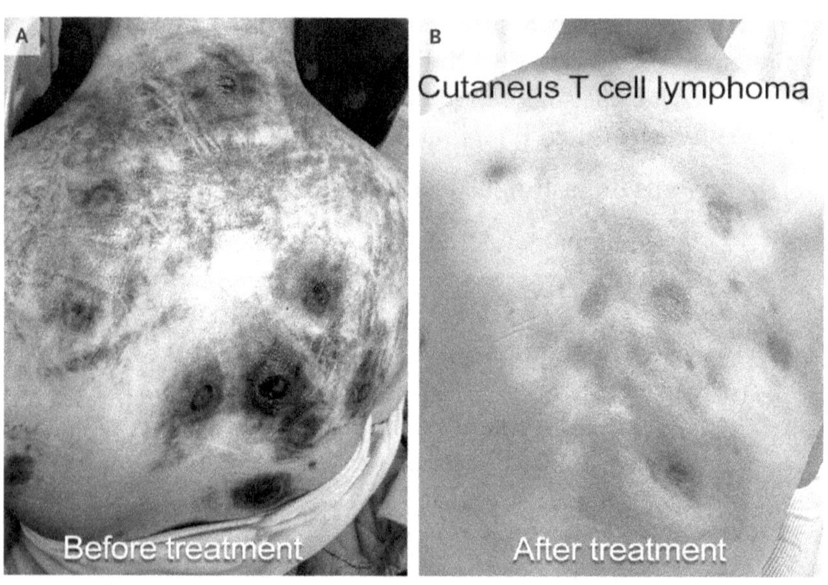

Bone and Bone Marrow

The primary involvement of the bone in NHL is classified as Stage 1 lymphoma, while the secondary involvement with widespread (disseminated) disease is considered Stage 4.

The vast majority of bone lymphomas are associated with NHL and caused by a type known as B-cell lymphoma. HL almost never affects the bone. □

When lymphoma affects the bone marrow, it can drastically impair the production of red and white blood cells, causing anemia (low red blood cells) and thrombocytopenia (low platelets). It also suppresses a specific white blood cell produced in the bone marrow called a leukocyte, leading to leukopenia. (Leukocytes are the same cells in involved in a related blood cancer known as leukemia.)

Symptoms of bone lymphoma include:

- Bone pain
- Limb swelling
- Loss of range of motion in a limb
- Fatigue
- Easy bruising and bleeding8□

If the spine is involved, lymphoma can cause numbness or tingling sensations in the arms or legs (peripheral neuropathy) as well as the loss of bladder or bowel control.

Central Nervous System

Lymphomas of the central nervous system (CNS) represent between 7% and 15% of all brain cancers. They are usually classified as B-cell lymphoma and occur most commonly in immunocompromised people, such as those with advanced HIV infection.

Symptoms of primary or secondary CNS lymphoma include:

- Headaches
- Muscle weakness in a specific body part
- Loss of sensation in a specific body part

- Problems with balance, memory, cognition, and/or language
- Changes in vision or partial vision loss
- Nausea and vomiting
- Seizures ☐

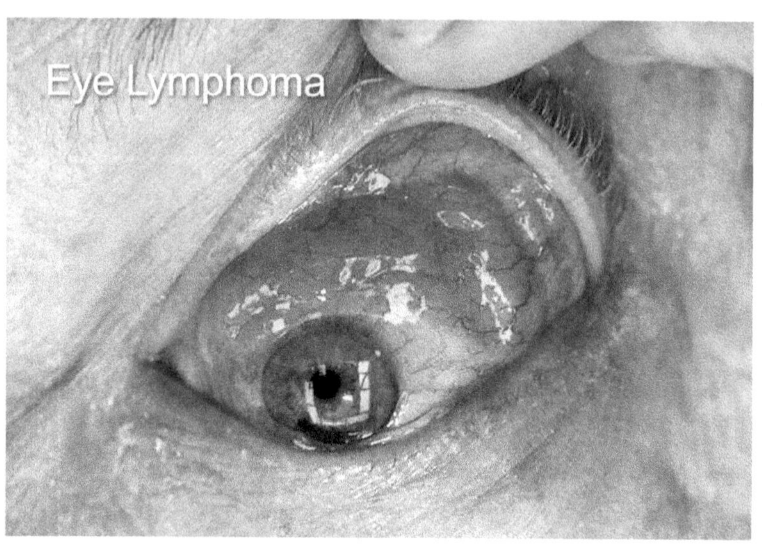

Lungs

Pulmonary (lung) lymphoma is more common with HL than NHL. With HL, it is secondary to the mediastinal lymph nodes of the chest. If it occurs with NHL, it is most often primary and caused by MALT lymphoma.

Symptoms of pulmonary lymphoma are often non-specific in the early stages of the disease and may include:

- Coughing
- Chest pain
- Fever
- Shortness of breath
- Crepitus (audible lung crackles)
- Hemoptysis (coughing up blood)
- Unintended weight loss □

With advanced pulmonary lymphoma, there may also be atelectasis (a collapsed lung) or pleural effusion ("water on the lungs"). By this stage of the disease, the lungs will usually not be the only organs involved.

Liver

Primary liver lymphoma is extremely rare and almost exclusively associated with NHL. With that said, there will be secondary liver involvement in 15% of people with NHL and 10% of those with NL. In most cases, the malignancy will have spread from the retroperitoneal lymph nodes situated to the back of the abdominal cavity to the liver.

Symptoms of liver lymphoma are often mild and non-specific and may include:

- Extreme fatigue
- Pain or swelling in the upper right abdomen
- Loss of appetite

- Nausea and vomiting
- Jaundice (yellowing of the skin and/or eyes)
- Dark urine
- Unintended weight loss☐

Kidneys and Adrenal Glands

As with the liver, primary lymphoma of the kidneys and adrenal glands is rare. Primary or secondary kidney lymphoma often mimics renal cell carcinoma, a type of cancer that starts in the small tubes of the kidney and causes symptoms such as:

- Flank pain
- A lump or swelling in the side or abdomen
- Hematuria (blood in urine)
- Loss of appetite
- Fever
- Persistent fatigue
- Unintended weight loss☐

Lymphoma of the adrenal glands will typically manifest with adrenal insufficiency, also known as Addison's disease.

Genitals

Testicular lymphoma accounts for around 5% of all abnormal growth in the testicles. It typically manifests with painless swelling, usually in one testicle only. What makes testicular lymphoma especially concerning is that it tends to involve aggressive B-cell lymphomas that move quickly into the central nervous system.

Genital involvement is women is rare, although cases involving the cervix and uterus have been reported. More often than not, women will experience lymphoma not in the genitals themselves but in tissues surrounding the genitals, known as the adnexa.

Complications

There are six different types of HL (including "classical" nodular sclerosing Hodgkin lymphoma) and over 60 types and subtypes of NHL (of which 85% are B-cell lymphomas).

The types and subtypes can be further differentiated by their grade, some of which will be low-grade (slow-growing) and others of which will be high-grade (aggressive). These characteristics can often predict how quickly and extensively symptoms will develop and progress.

Because lymphoma weakens the immune system, it can lead to serious long-term complications. This is especially true with low-grade lymphomas, many of which cannot be cured.

While modern therapies have afforded near-normal life expectancies in people with lymphoma, ongoing exposure to chemotherapy drugs may trigger the early development of aging-related diseases, such as cancer and heart disease.

Cancer

Secondary cancers, including leukemia and solid tumors, are among the leading causes of death in people with lymphoma. Leukemia can often develop years and even decades after exposure to alkylating chemotherapy drugs, while 70% to 80% of all secondary solid tumors occur in people with previous exposure to combined radiation and chemotherapy.

Breast cancer in women with HL often occurs 10 to 15 years after chest irradiation, particularly in those under 35. Similarly, lung cancer rates are higher in people with HL who are smokers and have previously undergone radiation and/or chemotherapy.

Higher doses of radiation confer to a greater risk of secondary breast or lung cancer, increasing the risk by as much as 900% greater compared to low-dose chest irradiation.

Heart Disease

Heart disease is believed to be the leading, non-cancer cause of death in people with lymphoma. Among the chief concerns is coronary artery disease (CAD), which occurs at a rate three- and five-times greater than that of the general population. Most CAD cases develop 10 to 25 years after exposure to chest radiation therapy for lymphoma.

Similarly, radiation to the neck is associated with a two- to five-fold increase in the risk of stroke. As with CAD, pre-existing heart disease, smoking, diabetes, and high blood pressure only adds to the risk.

Hormonal Disorders and Infertility

As a disease that often affects organs of the endocrine system, lymphoma may cause hormonal imbalances or insufficiencies that can persist for years following the successful treatment of the disease.

The most common complication is hypothyroidism (low thyroid function), affecting as many as 60% of people with HL. The risk is hypothyroidism is directly related to the amount of radiation used to treat the disease, particularly in advanced, late-stage lymphoma.

Infertility is a common concern in people with lymphoma. While testicular lymphoma can most certainly impact a man's fertility, the alkylating chemotherapy drugs used to treat lymphoma are the most common causes of infertility in both men and women.

People treated with the BEACOPP regimen of chemotherapy drugs (bleomycin, etoposide, doxorubicin, cyclophosphamide, procarbazine, and prednisone) were most severely affected.

As many as 50% of women treated with a BEACOPP chemotherapy will experience abnormal menstrual cycles, while 89% of men will develop azoospermia (the absence of motile sperm).

Other chemotherapy regimens (such as AVBD) are less impactful. By and large, men and women with chemotherapy-induced infertility will experience restored fertility after the completion of therapy, although some may end up experiencing permanent sterility.

Diagnosis

Most people with non-Hodgkin lymphoma (NHL) see their doctor because they have felt a lump that hasn't gone away, they develop some of the other symptoms of NHL, or they just don't feel well and go in for a check-up.

If you have signs or symptoms that suggest you might have lymphoma, exams and tests will be done to find out for sure and, if so, to determine the exact type of lymphoma.

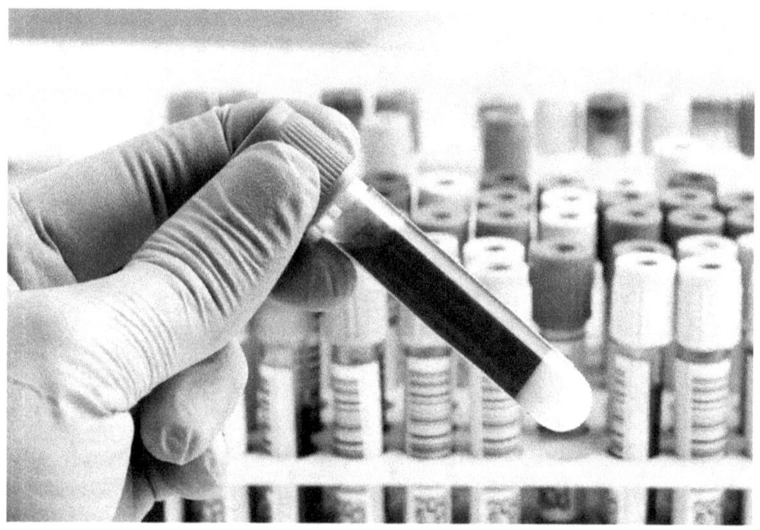

Medical history and physical exam

Your doctor will want to get a complete medical history, including information about your symptoms, possible risk factors, and other medical conditions.

Next, the doctor will examine you, paying special attention to the lymph nodes and other areas of the body that might be affected, including the spleen and liver. Because infections are the most common cause of enlarged lymph nodes, the doctor will look for an infection near the swollen lymph nodes.

The doctor also might order blood tests to look for signs of infection or other problems. Blood tests aren't used to diagnose lymphoma, though. If the doctor suspects that lymphoma might be causing your symptoms, he or she might recommend a biopsy of a swollen lymph node or other affected area.

Biopsy

For a biopsy, a small piece of a lymph node or, more often, an entire lymph node is removed for testing in a lab.

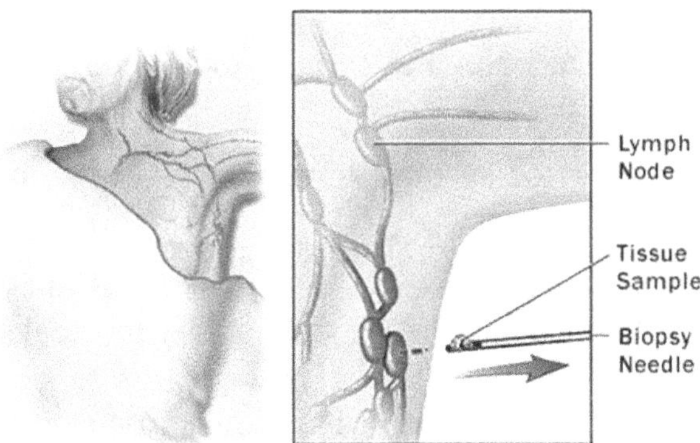

A biopsy is the only way to confirm a person has NHL. But it's not always done right away because many symptoms of NHL can also be caused by other problems, like an infection, or by other kinds of cancer. For example, enlarged lymph nodes are more often caused by infections than by lymphoma. Because of this, doctors often prescribe antibiotics and wait a few weeks to see if the lymph nodes shrink. If the nodes stay the same or continue to grow, the doctor might order a biopsy.A biopsy might be needed right away if the size, texture, or location of a lymph node or the presence of other symptoms strongly suggests lymphoma.

Biopsies to diagnose non-Hodgkin lymphoma

There are several types of biopsies. Doctors choose which one to use based on each person's situation.

Excisional or incisional biopsy

This is the preferred and most common type of biopsy if lymphoma is suspected, because it almost always provides enough of a sample to diagnose the exact type of NHL.

In this procedure, a surgeon cuts through the skin to remove the lymph node.

If the doctor removes the entire lymph node, it is called an excisional biopsy.

If a small part of a larger tumor or node is removed, it is called an incisional biopsy.

If the enlarged node is just under the skin, this is a fairly simple operation that can often be done with local anesthesia (numbing medicine). But if the node is inside the chest or abdomen, you will be sedated (given drugs to make you drowsy and relaxed) or given general anesthesia (drugs to put you into a deep sleep).

Needle biopsy

Needle biopsies are less invasive than excisional or incisional biopsies, but the drawback is that they might not remove enough of a sample to diagnose lymphoma (or to determine which type it is). Most doctors do not use needle biopsies to diagnose lymphoma. But if the doctor suspects that your lymph node is enlarged because of an infection or by the spread of cancer from another organ (such as the breast, lungs, or thyroid), a needle biopsy may be the first type of biopsy done. An excisional biopsy might still be needed even after a needle biopsy has been done, to diagnose and classify lymphoma.

There are 2 main types of needle biopsies:

In a **fine needle aspiration (FNA) biopsy**, the doctor uses a very thin, hollow needle attached to a syringe to withdraw (aspirate) a small amount of tissue from an enlarged lymph node or a tumor mass.

For a **core needle biopsy**, the doctor uses a larger needle to remove a slightly larger piece of tissue.

To biopsy an enlarged node just under the skin, the doctor can aim the needle while feeling the node. If the node or tumor is deep inside the body, the doctor can guide the needle using a computed tomography (CT) scan or ultrasound.

If lymphoma has already been diagnosed, needle biopsies are sometimes used to check abnormal areas in other parts of the body that might be from the lymphoma spreading or coming back after treatment.

Other types of biopsies

These procedures are not normally done to diagnose lymphoma, but they might be used to help determine the stage (extent) of a lymphoma that has already been diagnosed.

Bone marrow aspiration and biopsy

These procedures are often done after lymphoma has been diagnosed to help determine if it has reached the bone marrow. The 2 tests are often done at the same time. The samples are usually taken from the back of the pelvic (hip) bone, although in some cases they may be taken from other bones.

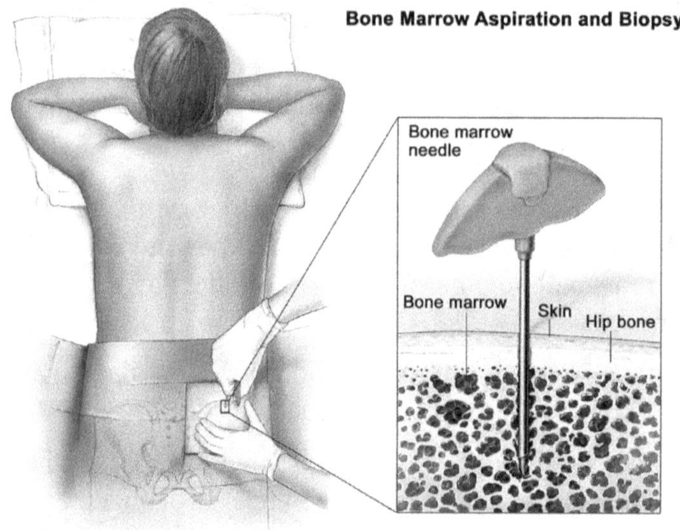

For a bone marrow aspiration, you lie on a table (either on your side or on your belly). After cleaning the skin over the hip, the doctor numbs the area and the surface of the bone with local anesthetic, which can cause a brief stinging or burning sensation. A thin, hollow needle is then inserted into the bone and a syringe is used to suck out a small amount of liquid bone marrow. Even with the anesthetic, most people still have some brief pain when the marrow is removed.

A bone marrow biopsy is usually done just after the aspiration. A small piece of bone and marrow is removed with a slightly larger needle that is pushed into the bone. The biopsy can also cause some brief pain.

Lumbar puncture (spinal tap)

This test looks for lymphoma cells in the cerebrospinal fluid (CSF), which is the liquid that bathes the brain and spinal cord.

Most people with lymphoma will not need this test. But doctors may order it for certain types of lymphoma or if a person has symptoms that suggest the lymphoma may have reached the brain.

For this test, you may lie on your side or sit up. The doctor first numbs an area in the lower part of your back over the spine. A small, hollow needle is then placed between the bones of the spine to withdraw some of the fluid.

Pleural or peritoneal fluid sampling

Lymphoma that has spread to the chest or abdomen can cause fluid to build up. Pleural fluid (inside the chest) or peritoneal fluid (inside the abdomen) can be removed by placing a hollow needle through the skin into the chest or abdomen.

When this procedure is used to remove fluid from the area around the lung, it's called a **thoracentesis**.

When it is used to collect fluid from inside the abdomen, it's known as a **paracentesis**.

The doctor uses a local anesthetic to numb the skin before inserting the needle. The fluid is then taken out and checked in the lab for lymphoma cells.

Lab tests on biopsy samples

All biopsy samples and fluids are looked at in the lab by a pathologist (a doctor specially trained to recognize cancer cells). The size and shape of the cells and how they are arranged may show not only if the person has a lymphoma, but also what type of lymphoma it is. But usually other types of lab tests are needed as well.

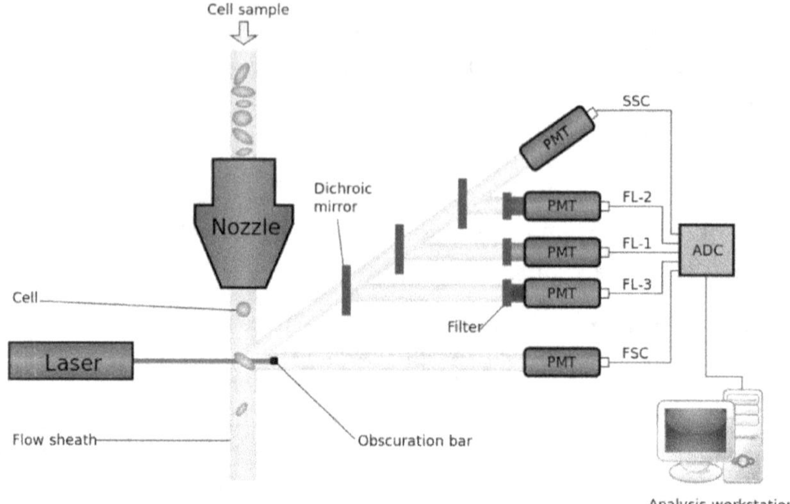

Flow cytometry and immunohistochemistry

For both flow cytometry and immunohistochemistry, the biopsy samples are treated with antibodies that stick to certain proteins on cells. The cells are then looked at in the lab (immunohistochemistry) or with a special machine (for flow cytometry), to see if the antibodies attached to them.

These tests can help determine whether a lymph node is swollen because of lymphoma, some other cancer, or a non-cancerous disease. The tests can also be used for immunophenotyping – determining which type of lymphoma a person has, based on certain proteins in or on the cells. Different types of lymphocytes have different proteins on their surface, which correspond to the type of lymphocyte and how mature it is.

Chromosome tests

Normal human cells have 23 pairs of chromosomes (strands of DNA), each of which is a certain size and looks a certain way in the lab. But in some types of lymphoma, the cells have changes in their chromosomes, such as having too many, too few, or abnormal chromosomes. These changes can often help identify the type of lymphoma.

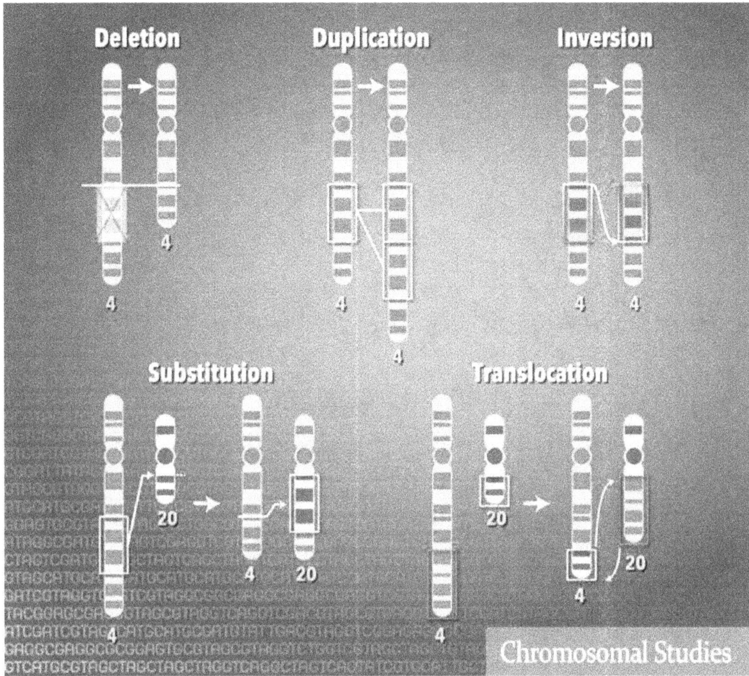

Cytogenetics

In this lab test, the cells are checked for any abnormalities in the chromosomes.

Fluorescent in situ hybridization (FISH)

This test looks more closely at lymphoma cell DNA using special fluorescent dyes that only attach to specific genes or parts of chromosomes. FISH can find most chromosome changes that can be seen in standard cytogenetic tests, as well as some gene changes too small to be seen with cytogenetic testing. FISH is very accurate and can usually provide results within a couple of days.

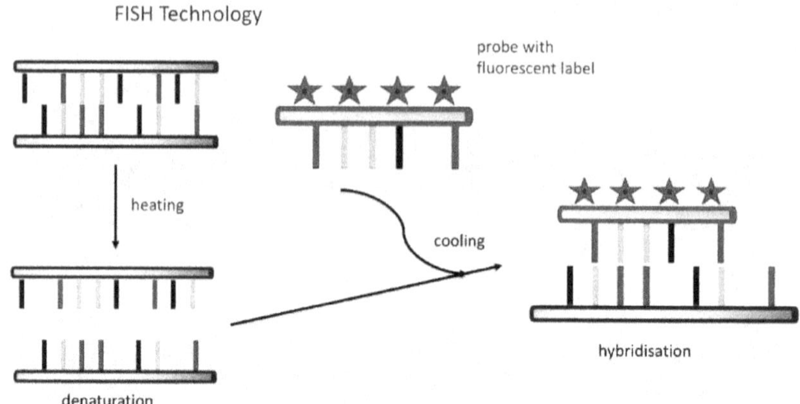

Polymerase chain reaction (PCR): PCR is a very sensitive DNA test that can find gene changes and certain chromosome changes too small to be seen with a microscope, even if very few lymphoma cells are present in a sample.

Imaging tests

Imaging tests use x-rays, ultra sound waves, magnetic fields, or radioactive particles to produce pictures of the inside of the body. These tests might be done for a number of reasons, including:

- To look for possible causes of certain symptoms (such as enlarged lymph nodes in the chest in someone having chest pain or trouble breathing)
- To help determine the stage (extent) of the lymphoma
- To help show if treatment is working
- To look for possible signs of lymphoma coming back after treatment

Chest x-ray

The chest might be x-rayed to look for enlarged lymph nodes in this area.

Computed tomography (CT) scan

A CT scan combines many x-rays to make detailed, cross-sectional images of your body. This scan can help tell if any lymph nodes or organs in your body are enlarged. CT scans are useful for looking for lymphoma in the abdomen, pelvis, chest, head, and neck.

CT-guided needle biopsy A CT can also be used to guide a biopsy needle into a suspicious area. For this procedure, you lie on the CT scanning table while the doctor moves a biopsy needle through the skin and toward the area. CT scans are repeated until the needle is in the right place. A biopsy sample is then removed to be looked at in the lab.

Magnetic resonance imaging (MRI) scan

Like CT scans, MRI scans show detailed images of soft tissues in the body. But MRI scans use radio waves and strong magnets instead of x-rays. This test is not used as often as CT scans for lymphoma, but if your doctor is concerned about spread to the spinal cord or brain, MRI is very useful for looking at these areas.

Ultrasound

Ultrasound uses sound waves and their echoes to create pictures of internal organs or masses. In the most common type of ultrasound, a small, microphone-like instrument called a transducer is placed on the skin (which is first lubricated with a gel). It gives off sound waves and picks up the echoes as they bounce off the organs. The echoes are converted by a computer into an image on a computer screen.

Ultrasound can be used to look at lymph nodes near the surface of the body or to look inside your abdomen for enlarged lymph nodes or organs such as the liver and spleen. It can also detect kidneys that have become swollen because the outflow of urine has been blocked by enlarged lymph nodes.

Positron emission tomography (PET) scan

For a PET scan, you are injected with a slightly radioactive form of sugar, which collects mainly in cancer cells. A special camera is then used to create a picture of areas of radioactivity in the body. The picture is not detailed like a CT or MRI scan, but it can provide helpful information about your whole body.

If you have lymphoma, a PET scan might be done to:

- See if an enlarged lymph node contains lymphoma.
- Find small areas that might be lymphoma, even if the area looks normal on a CT scan.
- Check if a lymphoma is responding to treatment. Some doctors will repeat the PET scan after 1 or 2 courses of chemotherapy. If the chemotherapy is working, the lymph nodes will no longer absorb the radioactive sugar.
- Help decide whether an enlarged lymph node still contains lymphoma or is just scar tissue after treatment.

PET/CT scan

Some machines can do both a PET scan and a CT scan at the same time. This lets the doctor compare areas of higher radioactivity on the PET scan with the more detailed appearance of that area on the CT scan. PET/CT scans can often help pinpoint the areas of lymphoma better than a CT scan alone.

Bone scan

This test is usually done if a person is having bone pain or has lab results that suggest the lymphoma may have reached the bones.

For bone scans, a radioactive substance called technetium is injected into a vein. It travels to damaged areas of bone, and a special camera can then detect the radioactivity. Lymphoma often causes bone damage, which may be seen on a bone scan. But bone scans can't show the difference between cancers and non-cancerous problems, such as arthritis and fractures, so further tests might be needed.

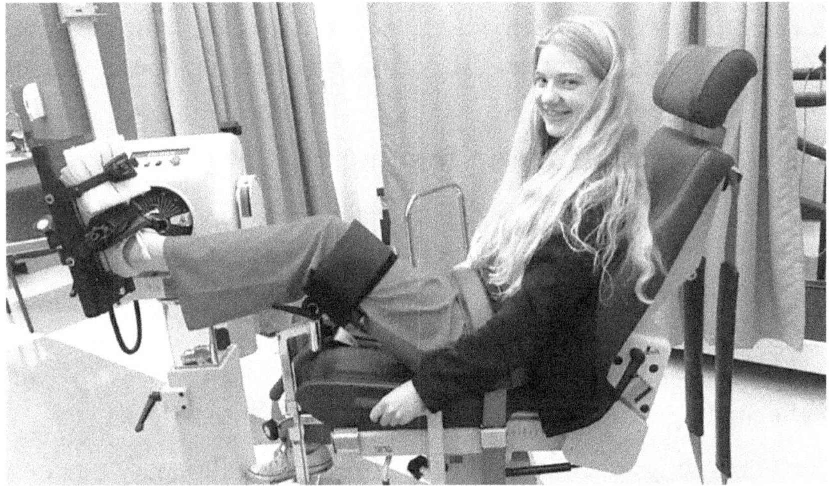

Blood tests

Blood tests are not used to diagnose lymphoma, but they can sometimes help determine how advanced the lymphoma is.

A complete blood count (CBC) measures the levels of different cells in the blood. For a person already known to have lymphoma, low blood cell counts might mean that the lymphoma is growing in the bone marrow and affecting new blood cell formation.

Blood chemistry tests are often done to look at how well the kidney and liver function are working.

If lymphoma has been diagnosed, **the lactate dehydrogenase (LDH) level** may be checked. LDH levels are often increased in patients with lymphomas.

For some types of lymphoma or if certain treatments might be used, your doctor may also advise you to have tests to see if you've been infected with certain viruses, such as **hepatitis B virus (HBV), hepatitis C virus (HCV), or human immunodeficiency virus (HIV)**. Infections with these viruses may affect your treatment.

Tests of heart and lung function

These tests are not used to diagnose lymphoma, but they might be done if you are going to get certain chemotherapy drugs commonly used to treat lymphoma that could affect the heart or the lungs.

Your heart function may be checked with an **echocardiogram** (an ultrasound of the heart) or a **MUGA** scan.

Your lung function may be checked with pulmonary function tests, in which you breathe into a tube connected to a machine.

Non-Hodgkin Lymphoma Stages

After someone is diagnosed with Non-Hodgkin Lymphoma, doctors will try to figure out if it has spread, and if so, how far. This process is called staging. The stage of a cancer describes how much cancer is in the body. It helps determine how serious the cancer is and how best to treat it. .

Tests used to gather information for staging can include:

- Physical exam
- Biopsies of enlarged lymph nodes or other abnormal areas
- Blood tests
- Imaging tests, such as PET and CT scans
- Bone marrow aspiration and biopsy (often but not always done)
- Lumbar puncture (spinal tap – this may not need to be done)

In general, the results of imaging tests such as PET or CT scans are the most important when determining the stage of the lymphoma.

Lugano classification

A staging system is a way for members of a cancer care team to sum up the extent of a cancer's spread. The current staging system for NHL in adults is known as the Lugano classification, which is based on the older Ann Arbor system.

The stages are described by Roman numerals I through IV (1-4). Limited stage (I or II) lymphomas that affect an organ outside the lymph system (an extranodal organ) have an E added (for example, stage IIE).

Stage I

Either of the following means the disease is stage I:

The lymphoma is in only 1 lymph node area or lymphoid organ such as the tonsils (I).

The cancer is found only in 1 area of a single organ outside of the lymph system (IE).

Stage II

Either of the following means the disease is stage II:

The lymphoma is in 2 or more groups of lymph nodes on the same side of (above or below) the diaphragm (the thin band of muscle that separates the chest and abdomen). For example, this might include nodes in the underarm and neck area (II) but not the combination of underarm and groin nodes (III).

The lymphoma is in a group of lymph node(s) and in one area of a nearby organ (IIE). It may also affect other groups of lymph nodes on the same side of the diaphragm.

Stage III

Either of the following means the disease is stage III:

The lymphoma is in lymph node areas on both sides of (above and below) the diaphragm.

The lymphoma is in lymph nodes above the diaphragm, as well as in the spleen.

Stage IV

The lymphoma has spread widely into at least one organ outside the lymph system, such as the bone marrow, liver, or lung.

Bulky disease

This term is often used to describe large tumors in the chest. It is especially important for stage II lymphomas, as bulky disease might need more intensive treatment.

Staging small lymphocytic lymphoma (SLL)/chronic lymphocytic leukemia (CLL)

The system above is most often used to stage this lymphoma if it is only in lymph nodes. But if the disease is affecting the blood or bone marrow, it is often staged using the systems for CLL.

How staging might affect treatment

The stage of a lymphoma is important when determining a person's treatment options, but it is more important for some types of lymphoma than for others. For many of the more common types of NHL, treatment is based in part on whether the lymphoma is "limited" (stage I or stage II non-bulky) or "advanced" (stage III or IV). For stage II bulky lymphomas, certain other factors (known as prognostic factors) are used to help determine if the lymphoma should be treated as limited or advanced.

For some other types of NHL, such as fast-growing lymphomas like Burkitt lymphoma, the stage is less important when deciding on treatment.

Differential Diagnosis

Because the signs and symptoms of lymphoma are subtle in the early stages, they are easily mistaken for other diseases. Even with advanced-stage extranodal lymphoma (lymphoma occurring outside of the lymphatic system), the symptoms can vary dramatically based on which organ is affected. Oftentimes, the disease will only be diagnosed when multiple extranodal sites are involved.

When diagnosing lymphoma, your doctor will want to rule out any other possible cause, particularly if the results of your biopsy are inconclusive. These may include:

- Bacteria infections like syphilis and tuberculosis

- Viral infections like HIV, cytomegalovirus, hepatitis B, hepatitis C, and Epstein-Barr virus (infectious mononucleosis)

- Parasitic infections like toxoplasmosis and leishmaniasis

- Autoimmune disorders like lupus and Sjogren's syndrome

- Cancers such as renal cell carcinoma (kidney cancer), squamous cell carcinoma of the lungs, melanoma (skin cancer), and hepatocellular carcinoma (liver cancer)

- Granulomatous disorders like sarcoidosis and lymphomatoid granulomatosis

- Rare disorders like Castleman's disease (giant lymph node hyperplasia)

NHL Lymphoma Treatment

To someone newly diagnosed with lymphoma, the treatment options may be difficult to understand. There are nearly 30 different types of lymphoma, numerous subtypes, and a variety of disease stages, each of which requires different treatment approaches.

The two main types, Hodgkin lymphoma (HL) and non-Hodgkin lymphoma (NHL), may involve chemotherapy, radiation therapy, immunotherapy, or a combination of therapies. People with NHL may also benefit from newer biologic drugs and CAR T-cell therapy. Stem cell transplants are sometimes needed if lymphoma relapse occurs.

Not all lymphomas can be cured. Of the two main types, HL tends to be the most treatable. Certain aggressive forms of NHL can also be cured with aggressive chemotherapy. By contrast, indolent (slow-growing) NHL is not curable, although it can be managed successfully for years and even decades. Many indolent lymphomas may not even require treatment until there are overt signs of disease progression.

The response to treatment can also change over time. Treatments that once kept the disease under control may suddenly become ineffective, making it necessary to keep abreast of new and experimental therapies.

Active Surveillance

Many low-grade lymphomas remain indolent for years. Rather than exposing you to drugs that are likely to cause side effects, your doctor may recommend the active monitoring of the disease, also known as a "watch-and-wait" approach.

On average, people with indolent lymphoma live just as long if they delay therapy compared to those who start treatment immediately. If you have mild symptoms you can cope with, it is often better to reserve treatment until the lymphoma symptoms are harder to manage.

Active surveillance is commonly used for certain types of indolent NHL, including follicular lymphoma, marginal cell lymphoma (including MALT lymphoma), small lymphocytic lymphoma, Waldenström's macroglobulinemia, and mantle cell lymphoma.

Active surveillance is sometimes used for a form of HL, known as nodular lymphocyte-predominant Hodgkin lymphoma (NLPHL), once the affected lymph nodes have been surgically removed.

Active monitoring requires regular follow-up visits with your doctor, typically every two months for the first year and every three to six months thereafter.

Chemotherapy

Chemotherapy involves the use of cytotoxic (cell-killing) drugs that can halt the spread of cancer cells. Chemotherapy is usually prescribed when the disease is systemic, meaning that the cancer has spread throughout the body. The advantage of chemotherapy is that it can travel throughout the bloodstream to kill cancer cells wherever they are located.

Lymphoma is caused by the uncontrolled growth in one of two different types of white blood cells, known as T-cells and B-cells. The various drugs are tailored based on the type of lymphoma type you have as well as the stage of disease (ranging from stage 1 to stage 4).

Side effects of chemotherapy vary by the type of drug used and may include fatigue, nausea, vomiting, hair loss, mouth sores, changes in taste, and an increased risk of infection.

Radiation Therapy

Radiation therapy, also known as radiotherapy, uses high-energy X-rays to kill cancer cells and shrink tumors. Radiation is a local therapy, which means that it only affects cancer cells in the treated area.

Radiation is often used on its own to treat lymphomas that have not spread. These include nodal lymphomas (those occurring within the lymphatic system) and extranodal lymphomas (those occurring outside of the lymphatic system). In other cases, radiation will be combined with chemotherapy.

Radiation treatment is generally confined to the lymph nodes and surrounding tissues, a procedure referred to as involved-field radiation therapy (IFRT). If the lymphoma is extranodal, the radiation will be focused on tissues from which the cancer originated (known as the primary tumor site). In rare cases, extended field radiation (EFR) may be used to treat lymphoma that is widespread (although it is far less commonly used today than it once was).

The indications for radiation vary by the type and stage and stage:

HL is typically treated with radiation alone as long as the malignancy is localized. Advanced HL (stages 2B, 3, and 4) usually require chemotherapy with or without radiation.

Low-grade NHL (stages 1 and 2) tends to respond well to radiation. Advanced NHL typically requires aggressive CHOP or R-CHOP chemotherapy with or without radiation.

Lymphoma that has spread to the brain, spinal cord, or other organs may require radiation to alleviate pain and other symptoms (referred to as palliative radiotherapy).

Radiotherapy is delivered externally from a machine using a highly focused beam of photons, protons, or ions. Referred to as external beam radiation, the dose and target of radiation will be determined by a specialist known as a radiation oncologist.

Radiation treatments are typically given five days a week for several weeks. The procedure itself is painless and lasts only a few minutes. Common side effects include fatigue, skin redness, and blistering.

Radiation to the abdomen can cause nausea, diarrhea, and vomiting. Radiation to the lymph nodes of the neck may cause mouth dryness, mouth sores, hair loss, and difficulty swallowing.

Chemotherapy

Chemotherapy (chemo) is the use of anti-cancer drugs that are usually injected into a vein (IV) or taken by mouth. These drugs enter the bloodstream and reach almost all areas of the body, making this treatment very useful for lymphoma.

When might chemo be used?

Chemo is the main treatment for most people with non-Hodgkin lymphoma (NHL). Depending on the type and the stage of the lymphoma, chemo may be used alone or combined with other treatments, such as immunotherapy drugs or radiation therapy.

Which chemo drugs are used to treat non-Hodgkin lymphoma?

Many chemo drugs are useful in treating lymphoma. Often, several drugs are combined. The number of drugs, their doses, and the length of treatment depend on the type and stage of the lymphoma. Here are some of the drugs more commonly used to treat lymphoma (divided into groups based on how they work):

Alkylating agents

- Cyclophosphamide
- Chlorambucil
- Bendamustine
- Ifosfamide

Corticosteroids

- Prednisone
- Dexamethasone

Platinum drugs

- Cisplatin
- Carboplatin
- Oxaliplatin
- Purine analogs
- Fludarabine
- Pentostatin
- Cladribine (2-CdA)

Anti-metabolites

- Cytarabine (ara-C)
- Gemcitabine
- Methotrexate
- Pralatrexate

Anthracyclines

- Doxorubicin (Adriamycin)
- Liposomal doxorubicin (Caelyx)

Others

- Vincristine

- Mitoxantrone
- Etoposide (VP-16)
- Bleomycin

Chemo is often combined with an immunotherapy drug, especially rituximab (Rituxan).

Doctors give chemo in cycles, in which a period of treatment is followed by a period of rest to allow the body time to recover. Each chemo cycle generally lasts for several weeks. Most chemo treatments are given on an outpatient basis (in the doctor's office or clinic or hospital outpatient department), but some might require a hospital stay.

Sometimes a patient may get one chemo combination for several cycles and later switch to a different one if the first combination doesn't seem to be working.

There are a number of standard chemotherapy regimens used in the United States:

ABVD regimen is used to treat all stages of HL. It involves the drugs Adriamycin (doxorubicin), Blenoxame (bleomycin), Velban (vinblastine), and DTIC (dacarbazine), which are delivered intravenously (into a vein) in four-week cycles. Depending on the disease stage, anywhere from one to eight cycles may be needed.

BEACOPP regimen may be prescribed to treat aggressive forms of HL using a combination of intravenous (IV) and oral drugs. BEACOPP stands for bleomycin, etoposide, doxorubicin, cyclophosphamide, Oncovin (vincristine), procarbazine, and prednisone. Treatment typically involves six to eight 21-day cycles.

CHOP regimen is used to treat both indolent and aggressive NHL types. CHOP is an acronym for cyclophosphamide, hydroxydaunomycin (a.k.a. doxorubicin),

Oncovin, and prednisone. The drugs, some of which are delivered by IV and others by mouth, are given in six to eight 21-day cycles.

R-CHOP regimen is used to treat diffuse large B cell lymphoma (DLBCL) and involves an additional biologic drug known as Rituxan (rituximab). It is also delivered in six to eight 21-day cycles.

Most of these chemotherapy drugs have been in use for decades. In recent years, newer agents have been developed that appear to be extremely effective and offer fewer side effects.

Newer chemotherapy drugs include Treanda (bendamustine), an intravenous drug used for people with indolent B-cell lymphoma and the injectable drug Folotyn (pralatrexate) used for those with relapsed or treatment-resistant T-cell lymphoma.

There are other combinations used to treat specific types of lymphoma, known by such acronyms as CVP, DHAP, and DICE. Other are used in combination with immunotherapy drugs that are not directly cytotoxic but spur the immune system to kill cancer cells.

Intrathecal chemo

Most chemo drugs given systemically (IV or by mouth) can't reach the cerebrospinal fluid (CSF) and tissues around the brain and spinal cord. To treat lymphoma that might have reached these areas, chemo may also be given into the CSF. This is called intrathecal chemo. The chemo drugs most often used for intrathecal chemo are methotrexate and cytarabine.

Possible side effects

Chemo drugs can cause side effects. These depend on the type and dose of drugs given and how long treatment lasts. Common side effects can include:

- Hair loss
- Mouth sores
- Loss of appetite
- Nausea and vomiting
- Diarrhea or constipation
- Increased chance of infection (from a shortage of white blood cells)
- Bleeding or bruising after minor cuts or injuries (from a shortage of platelets)
- Fatigue and shortness of breath (from too few red blood cells)

These side effects usually go away after treatment is finished. If serious side effects occur, the dose of chemo may be reduced or treatment may be delayed.

There are often ways to lessen these side effects. For example, drugs can be given to prevent or reduce nausea and vomiting.

Certain chemo drugs can have other possible side effects. For example:

Platinum drugs such as cisplatin can cause nerve damage (neuropathy), leading to numbness, tingling, or even pain in the hands and feet.

Ifosfamide can damage the bladder. The risk of this can be lowered by giving it along with a drug called mesna.

Doxorubicin can damage the heart. Your doctor may order a test of your heart function (like a MUGA scan or echocardiogram) before starting you on this drug.

Bleomycin can damage lungs. Doctors often test lung function before starting someone on this drug.

Many chemo drugs can affect fertility (the ability to have children).

Some chemo drugs can raise your risk of developing leukemia several years later.

Tumor lysis syndrome is a possible side effect when chemo is started, especially in patients with large or fast-growing lymphomas. Killing the lymphoma cells releases their contents into the bloodstream. This can overwhelm the kidneys, which can't get rid of all of these substances at once. This can lead to the build-up of certain minerals in the blood and even kidney failure. The excess minerals can lead to heart and nervous system problems. Doctors work to prevent this by giving the patient extra fluids and certain drugs, such as sodium bicarbonate, allopurinol, and rasburicase.

Ask your health care team about what side effects you can expect based on the specific drugs you will receive. Be sure to tell your doctor or nurse if you do have side effects, as there are often ways to help with them. For example, drugs can be given to prevent or reduce nausea and vomiting.

Other drugs used to treat lymphoma

Other types of drugs can also be useful in treating some types of lymphoma. These drugs work differently from standard chemo drugs. For example, immunotherapy and targeted therapy drugs are helpful for some lymphomas.

Mucosa-associated lymphoid tissue (MALT) lymphoma, which usually starts in the stomach, is linked to infection with the bacterium H. pylori. Treatment of this infection can often make the lymphoma go away. This is most often done with a combination of antibiotics along with drugs called proton pump inhibitors, which lower stomach acid levels.

In a similar way, splenic marginal zone B-cell lymphoma is sometimes linked to infection with the hepatitis C virus. Treating the infection with anti-viral drugs can sometimes shrink these lymphomas, or even make them go away.

Immunotherapy for NHL

Immunotherapy is treatment that either boosts the patient's own immune system or uses man-made versions of the normal parts of the immune system to kill lymphoma cells or slow their growth.

Monoclonal antibodies

Antibodies are proteins made by your immune system to help fight infections. Man-made versions, called monoclonal antibodies, can be designed to attack a specific target, such as a substance on the surface of lymphocytes (the cells in which lymphomas start).

Several monoclonal antibodies are now used to treat non-Hodgkin lymphoma (NHL).

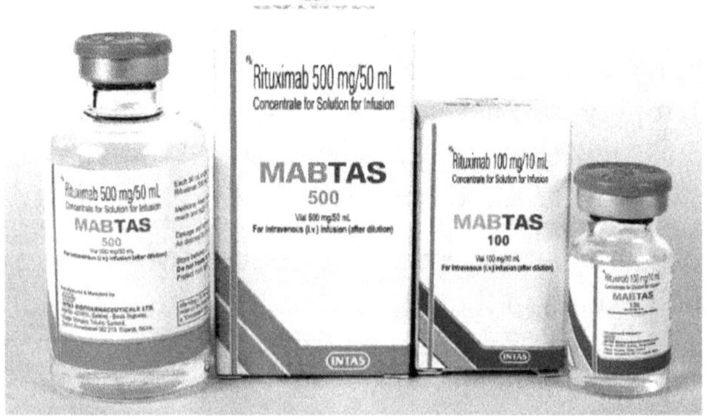

Antibodies that target CD20

A number of monoclonal antibodies target the CD20 antigen, a protein on the surface of B lymphocytes. These include:

Rituximab (Rituxan) This drug is often used along with chemotherapy (chemo) for some types of NHL, but it may also be used by itself.

Obinutuzumab (Gazyva) This drug is often used along with chemo as a part of the treatment for small lymphocytic lymphoma/chronic lymphocytic leukemia (SLL/CLL). It can also be used along with chemo in treating follicular lymphoma.

Ofatumumab (Arzerra): This drug is used mainly in patients with SLL/CLL that is no longer responding to other treatments.

Ibritumomab tiuxetan (Zevalin): This drug is made up of a monoclonal antibody that is attached to a radioactive molecule. The antibody brings radiation directly to the lymphoma cells.

These drugs are given into a vein (IV), often over several hours. They all can cause reactions during the infusion (while the drug is being given) or several hours afterward. Most reactions are mild, such as itching, chills, fever, nausea, rashes, fatigue, and headaches. More serious reactions can include chest pain, heart racing, swelling of the face and tongue, cough, trouble breathing, feeling dizzy or lightheaded, and feeling faint. Because of these kinds of reactions, drugs to help prevent them are given before each infusion.

There is also a form of rituximab that is given as a shot under the skin. It can take 5-7 minutes to inject the drug, but this is much shorter than the time it normally takes to give the drug by vein. It is approved for use in patients with follicular lymphoma, diffuse large B-cell lymphoma, and chronic lymphocytic leukemia. Possible side effects include local skin reactions, like redness, where the drug is injected, infections, low white blood cell counts, nausea, fatigue, and constipation.

All of these drugs can cause inactive hepatitis B infections to become active again, which can lead to severe or life-threatening liver problems. Your doctor may check your blood for signs of an old hepatitis B infection before you start treatment. These drugs can also increase your risk of certain serious infections for many months after the drug is stopped. Other side effects can depend on which drug is given. Ask your doctor what you can expect.

Antibodies targeting CD52

Alemtuzumab (Campath) is an antibody directed at the CD52 antigen. It is useful in some cases of SLL/CLL and some types of peripheral T-cell lymphomas. This drug is infused into a vein (IV), usually 3 times a week for up to 12 weeks. The most common side effects are fever, chills, nausea, and rashes. It can also cause very low white blood cell counts, which increases the risk for serious infections. Antibiotic and antiviral medicines are given to help protect against them, but severe and even life-threatening infections can still occur. Rare but serious side effects can include strokes, as well as tears in the blood vessels in the head and neck.

Antibodies that target CD30

Brentuximab vedotin (Adcetris) is an anti-CD30 antibody attached to a chemotherapy drug. The antibody acts like a homing signal, bringing the chemo drug to lymphoma cells, where it enters the cells and kills them.

Brentuximab can be used to treat some types of T-cell lymphoma, either as the first treatment (typically along with chemo) or if the lymphoma if it has come back after other treatments. This drug is infused into a vein (IV), typically every 3 weeks. Common side effects can include nerve damage (neuropathy), low blood counts, fatigue, fever, nausea and vomiting, infections, diarrhea, and cough.

Antibodies that target CD79b

Polatuzumab vedotin-piiq (Polivy) is an anti-CD79b antibody (polatuzumab) attached to a chemotherapy drug (MMAE). The antibody finds the lymphoma cell and attaches to the surface protein CD79b. Once connected, polatuzumab is drawn into the lymphoma cell where the chemo is released and destroys it.

Polatuzumab can be used with bendamustine and rituximab to treat DLBCL, if the lymphoma has come back after receiving two other treatments. This drug is infused into a vein (IV), typically every 3 weeks. Common side effects can include numbness or tingling of hands/feet (peripheral neuropathy), low blood counts, fatigue, fever, decreased appetite, diarrhea, and pneumonia.

Immune checkpoint inhibitors

Immune system cells normally have substances that act as checkpoints to keep them from attacking other healthy cells in the body. Cancer cells sometimes take advantage of these checkpoints to avoid being attacked by the immune system.

Drugs such as pembrolizumab (Keytruda) work by blocking these checkpoints, which can boost the immune response against cancer cells. Pembrolizumab can be used to treat primary mediastinal large B-cell lymphoma (PMBCL) that has not responded to or has come back after other therapies.

Immunomodulating drugs

Drugs such as thalidomide (Thalomid) and lenalidomide (Revlimid) are thought to work against certain cancers by affecting parts of the immune system, although exactly how they work isn't clear. They are sometimes used to help treat certain types of lymphoma, usually after other treatments have been tried. Lenalidomide can be given with or without rituximab.

These drugs are taken daily as pills. Side effects of can include low white blood cell counts (with an increased risk of infection) and neuropathy (painful nerve damage), which can sometimes be severe and may not go away after treatment. There is also an increased risk of serious blood clots (that start in the leg and can travel to the lungs), especially with thalidomide. Thalidomide can also cause drowsiness, fatigue, and severe constipation.

These drugs can cause severe birth defects if taken during pregnancy. Given this risk, the company that makes these drugs puts restrictions on access to them to prevent women who are or might become pregnant from being exposed to them.

Chimeric antigen receptor (CAR) T-cell therapy

In this treatment, immune cells called T cells are removed from the patient's blood and altered in the lab to have specific receptors (called chimeric antigen receptors, or CARs) on their surface. These receptors can attach to proteins on the surface of lymphoma cells. The T cells are then multiplied in the lab and given back into the patient's blood, where they can seek out the lymphoma cells and launch a precise immune attack against them.

Axicabtagene ciloleucel (Yescarta) is a type of CAR T-cell therapy approved by the FDA to treat people with diffuse large B-cell lymphoma, primary mediastinal large B-cell lymphoma, high grade B-cell lymphoma and diffuse large B-cell lymphoma arising from follicular lymphoma after at least two other kinds of treatment have been tried. Because this treatment can have serious side effects, it is only given in medical centers that have special training with this treatment. Potentially life-threatening side effects can include high fever, chills, flu-like symptoms, and serious neurological changes. Other severe side effects include infection, low blood cell counts, and a weakened immune system.

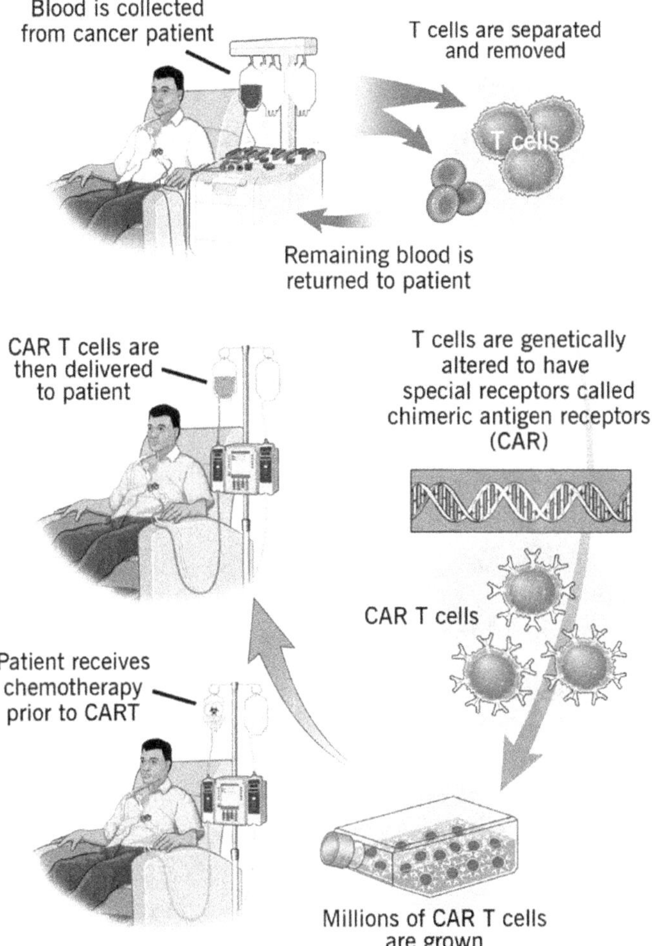

Tisagenlecleucel (Kymriah) is another type of CAR T-cell therapy approved to treat people with diffuse large B cell lymphoma, high grade B cell lymphoma, and diffuse large B cell lymphoma arising from follicular lymphoma after trying at least two other kinds of treatment. Potentially life-threatening side effects can include fever, headache, low blood pressure, a fast heart rate, and trouble breathing. Other severe side effects include infection, diarrhea, swelling, and nausea. This drug must also be given in centers with specialized training.

Targeted Therapy Drugs for NHL

As researchers have learned more about the changes in lymphoma cells that help them grow, they have developed newer drugs to specifically target these changes. These targeted drugs work differently from standard chemotherapy (chemo) drugs. Sometimes they work when standard chemo drugs don't, and they often have different (and less severe) side effects.

Proteasome inhibitors

These drugs work by stopping enzyme complexes (proteasomes) in cells from breaking down proteins important for keeping cell division under control. They are more often used to treat multiple myeloma, but can be helpful in treating some types of non-Hodgkin lymphoma (NHL) as well.

Bortezomib (Velcade) is a proteasome inhibitor used to treat some lymphomas, usually after other treatments have been tried. Bortezomib is given as an infusion into a vein (IV) or an injection under the skin (subcutaneous, or sub-q), typically twice a week for 2 weeks, followed by a rest period. Side effects can be similar to those of standard chemo drugs, including low blood counts, nausea, loss of appetite, and nerve damage.

Histone deacetylase (HDAC) inhibitors

HDAC inhibitors are drugs that can affect what genes are active by interacting with proteins in chromosomes called histones.

Romidepsin (Istodax) can be used to treat both peripheral and skin T-cell lymphomas. It is usually given after at least one other treatment has been tried. This drug is given as an IV infusion, usually once a week for 3 weeks in a row, followed by a week off. Side effects tend to be mild, but can include lowered blood cell counts and effects on heart rhythm.

Belinostat (Beleodaq) can be used to treat peripheral T-cell lymphomas, usually after at least one other treatment has been tried. It is given as an IV infusion, usually daily for 5 days in a row, repeated every 3 weeks. Common side effects include nausea, vomiting, tiredness, and low red blood cell counts (anemia).

Kinase inhibitors

These drugs block kinases, which are proteins in cells that normally relay signals (such as telling the cell to grow). Many different types of kinases exist, and there are two that are targeted by specific drugs used to treat NHL: Bruton's tyrosine kinase (BTK) and PI3K.

Bruton's tyrosine kinase (BTK) inhibitors

BTK is a protein that normally helps some lymphoma cells (B **cells) to grow and survive.**

Ibrutinib (Imbruvica) blocks the BTK protein. This drug can be used to treat several types of NHL, including mantle cell lymphoma, marginal zone lymphoma, and small lymphocytic lymphoma. It's taken by mouth as capsules, once a day. Common side effects include diarrhea or constipation, nausea and vomiting, fatigue, swelling, decreased appetite, and low blood counts. This drug is currently approved for use after other treatments have been tried, and it's now being studied for use earlier in treatment.

Acalabrutinib (Calquence) and zanubrutinib (Brukinsa) are other drugs that blocks BTK. They are used to treat mantle cell lymphoma, after at least one other treatment has been tried. These drugs are taken by mouth as capsules, twice a day. Common side effects are headache, diarrhea, bruising, fatigue, muscle pain, cough, rash, and low blood counts. More serious side effects can include bleeding (hemorrhage), infections, and irregular heartbeat (atrial fibrillation).

PI3K inhibitors

PI3K is a protein that sends signals in cells and controls cell growth.

Idelalisib (Zydelig) blocks the PI3K-delta protein. This drug has been shown to help treat follicular lymphoma and small lymphocytic lymphoma after other treatments have been tried. It's taken as a pill twice a day. Common side effects include diarrhea, fever, fatigue, nausea, cough, pneumonia, belly pain, chills, rash and low blood counts. Less often, more serious side effects can also occur.

Copanlisib (Aliqopa) is another drug that blocks PI3K. It can be used to treat follicular lymphoma that comes back after other treatments have been tried. It's given as an infusion into a vein, typically once a week for 3 weeks, followed by a week off. Common side effects include high blood sugar levels, nausea, diarrhea, feeling weak, high blood pressure, low levels of white blood cells (with increased risk of infection), and low levels of blood platelets (with increased risk of bruising or bleeding). Less common side effects include infections, inflammation in the lungs, and severe skin reactions.

Duvelisib (Copiktra) blocks two kinase proteins called PI3K-delta and PI3K-gamma. It's been shown to help treat follicular lymphoma and small lymphocytic lymphoma after other treatments have been tried. It's a pill taken twice a day.

Common side effects include diarrhea, fever, fatigue, nausea, cough, pneumonia, belly pain, joint/muscle pain and rash. Low blood counts, including low red blood cell counts (anemia) and low levels of certain white blood cells (neutropenia) are also common. Less often, more serious side effects can occur, such as liver damage, severe diarrhea, lung inflammation (pneumonitis), serious allergic reactions, severe skin problems.

Stem Cell Transplant

A stem cell transplant is a procedure that replaces damaged or destroyed stem cells in the bone marrow with healthy ones. It is typically used when a person has relapsed from intermediate- or high-grade lymphoma.

According to research published in Current Hematologic Malignancy Reports, 30% to 40% of people with NHL and 15% of those with HL will experience a relapse after the initial treatment.

Stem cells have the unique ability to transform into many different types of cells in the body. When used to treat lymphoma, the transplanted cells will stimulate the production of new blood cells. This is important since high-dose chemotherapy can damage bone marrow and impair the production of red and white blood cells needed to fight disease and function normally.

A stem cell transplant allows you to be treated with a higher dose of chemotherapy than you might otherwise be able to tolerate.

Before the transplant, high doses of chemotherapy (and sometimes radiation) are used to "condition" the body for the procedure. By doing so, the body is less likely to reject the stem cells. The conditioning process takes one to two weeks and is performed in a hospital due to the high risk of infection and side effects.

The main types of stem cell transplant used are:

Autologous transplantation uses a person's own stem cells which are harvested, treated, and returned to the body after the conditioning procedure.

Allogeneic transplantation uses stem cells from a donor. The cells can be taken from a family member or a non-related person.

Reduced-intensity stem cell transplantation is a form of allogeneic transplant that involves less chemotherapy (usually for older or sicker people).

Syngeneic transplantation is the type that occurs between identical twins who have identical genetic makeup.

Although the safety and effectiveness of stem cell transplant continue to improve every year, there are considerable risks. Not everyone is eligible for a transplant, particularly those unable to withstand the conditioning process. Moreover, the procedure does not work for people with tumors that are unresponsive to drugs.

Recovery from a stem cell transplant may take months to years and can permanently affect fertility. An in-depth consultation with a specialist oncologist is needed to fully weigh the benefits and risks of the procedure.

Prognosis

The prognosis of NHL can be good but depends on the type of lymphoma, the extent of spread (staging), and response to therapy. A health care provider will discuss the prognosis with the patient. The overall five-year survival rate for people with NHL is 71%, while the overall 10-year survival rate is 60%.

Five-year survival is a measure used to predict and gauge the severity of the cancer. Patients should discuss risk factors, staging, and classifications with their health care team as none of these numbers apply to an individual patient without considering all the circumstances of the patient's illness.

NHL Five-Year Survival

Stage at diagnosis	Stage distribution (%)	Five-year relative survival (%)
Localized (confined to primary site)	28	81.6
Regional (spread to regional lymph nodes)	15	72.9
Distant (cancer has metastasized)	49	61.6
Unknown (unstaged)	8	66.9

Hodgkin Lymphoma

Hodgkin lymphoma, also known as Morbus Hodgkin, Hodgkin's lymphoma or Hodgkin's Disease, is a cancer of the lymphatic system. Like the large entity of Non-Hodgkin-Lymphomas (NHL), it belongs to the group of malignant lymphomas.

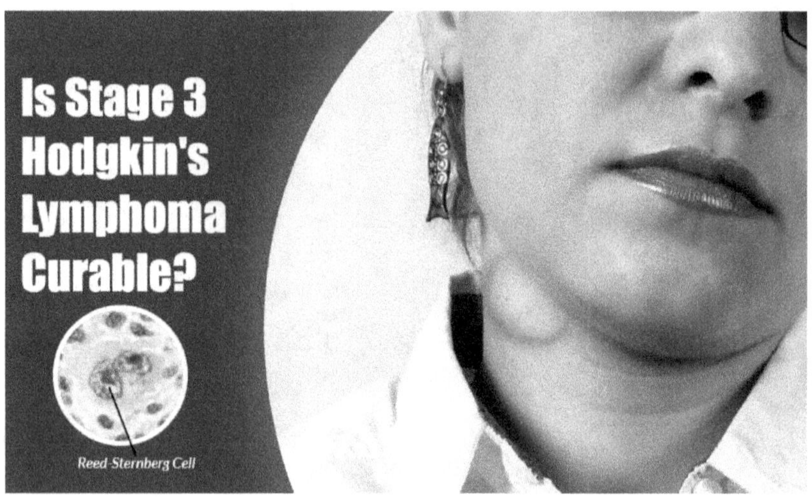

Hodgkin lymphoma develops from transformed B-lymphocytes, a type of white blood cells (leukocytes) found in lymphatic tissue. Hodgkin lymphoma can arise from every organ comprised of lymphatic tissue. The most common localisation is the lymph nodes, however, liver, bone marrow, lungs or spleen can also be affected, especially in advanced stages of the disease. Without adequate treatment, Hodgkin lymphoma is a fatal disease in most patients. Other names for Hodgkin lymphoma include Hodgkin's disease (HD) and Hodgkin's lymphoma.

Discovery and nomenclature history

Hodgkin lymphoma is named after Thomas Hodgkin (1798–1866), who was a physician from a Quaker family that studied medicine in Edinburgh and Paris. As one of the most prominent British pathologist of his time, he held the position of the conservator of the pathology museum at Guy's Hospital Medical School from 1825, where he studied preserved specimens of human organs.

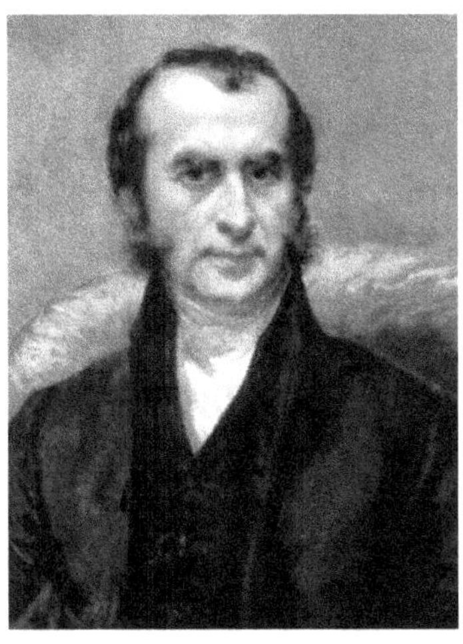

In 1832 he published a paper in the Journal of the Medical and Chirurgical Society in London entitled "On Some Morbid Appearances of the Absorbent Glands and Spleen" which went almost unnoticed at the time. More than three decades later, another British physician named Samuel Wilks described the same disease features and named the disease after Hodgkin. Since then this type of lymph node malignancy bears this name.

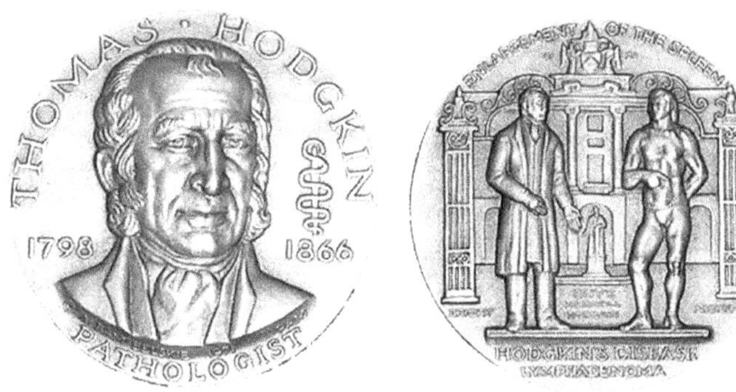

Incidence

Hodgkin lymphoma is the most frequent lymphoma disease in childhood. According to the German Childhood Cancer Registry in Mainz, about 80 children and teenagers aged younger than 15 are newly diagnosed with Hodgkin lymphoma in Germany per year. Depending on the age range considered, Hodgkin lymphoma accounts for approximately 4.5 % and 7.4 % of all paediatric malignancies, respectively.

Hodgkin lymphoma is rarely diagnosed in children younger than 3 years. With increasing age, incidence gets more and more frequent, with boys being slightly more affected than girls. The incidence in children and adolescents (between 0 and 17 years) peaks at 15 years of age.

Risk Factors

The exact cause of Hodgkin lymphoma is not known, but the following factors may raise a person's risk of developing Hodgkin lymphoma:

Age. People between the ages of 15 and 40 and people older than 55 are more likely to develop Hodgkin lymphoma.

Gender. In general, men are slightly more likely to develop Hodgkin lymphoma than women, although the nodular sclerosis subtype is more common in women.

Family history. Brothers and sisters of people with Hodgkin lymphoma have a higher chance of developing the disease, although the increase in risk is small.

Virus exposure. The Epstein-Barr virus (EBV) causes infectious mononucleosis, often called "mono." Nearly all adult Americans and many others around the world have an EBV infection. About 20% to 25% of people with cHL in the United

States have lymphoma cells that test positive for EBV. Although a person's immune system response to an infection with EBV may be important in the development of Hodgkin lymphoma, doctors still do not understand why, when so many people have been infected with EBV, relatively very few people ever develop Hodgkin lymphoma. People with HIV also have a higher risk of developing Hodgkin lymphoma, particularly lymphocyte-depleted Hodgkin lymphoma.

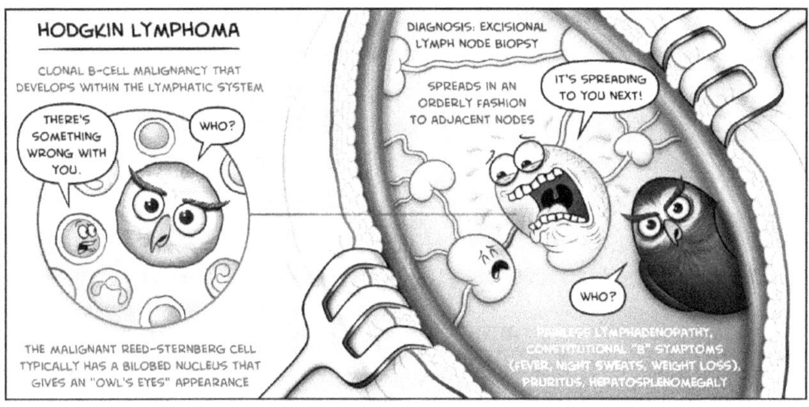

Types of Hodgkin lymphoma

There are different types of Hodgkin lymphoma. It is important to know the type because this may affect how the cancer is treated. Doctors determine the type of Hodgkin lymphoma based on how the cells look under a microscope and whether the cells contain certain abnormal proteins. These cells are taken using a tissue biopsy.

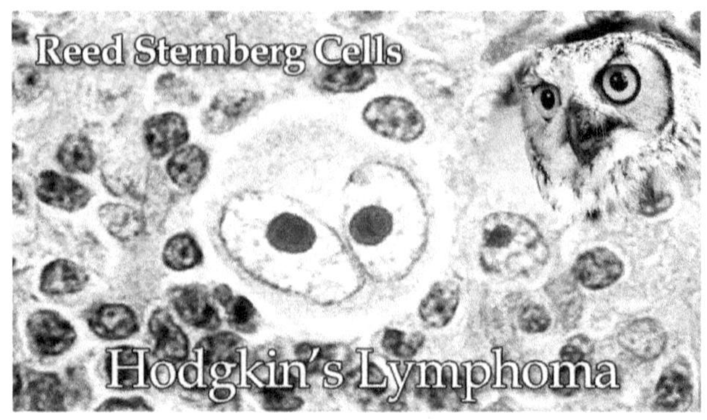

The American Joint Committee on Cancer (AJCC) recognizes 2 major categories of Hodgkin lymphoma: classic Hodgkin lymphoma, which is divided into 4 subtypes based on the appearance of the lymph node structure and cells, and nodular lymphocyte-predominant Hodgkin lymphoma.

Classic Hodgkin lymphoma (cHL)

cHL is the most common type of Hodgkin lymphoma. About 95% of cases of Hodgkin lymphoma are within the cHL category. cHL is diagnosed when characteristic abnormal lymphocytes, known as Reed-Sternberg cells, are found. cHL is divided into 4 subtypes:

Nodular sclerosis Hodgkin lymphoma Nodular sclerosis Hodgkin lymphoma is the most common subtype of cHL. It affects up to 80% of people diagnosed with cHL. Nodular sclerosis Hodgkin lymphoma is most common in young adults, especially women. In addition to Reed-Sternberg cells, there are bands of connective tissue (called fibrosis) found in the lymph node. The presence of these bands can help diagnose this type of Hodgkin lymphoma. This type of lymphoma often affects the lymph nodes in the central part of the chest, called the mediastinum.

Lymphocyte-rich classic Hodgkin lymphoma

About 6% of people with cHL are diagnosed with lymphocyte-rich classic Hodgkin lymphoma. It is more common in men and usually affects areas other than the mediastinum. In addition to Reed-Sternberg cells, the lymph node tissue contains many normal lymphocytes.

Mixed cellularity Hodgkin lymphoma This subtype of cHL occurs most often in older adults. It sometimes develops in the abdomen and carries many different cell types, including large numbers of Reed-Sternberg cells.

Lymphocyte-depleted Hodgkin lymphoma

Lymphocyte-depleted Hodgkin lymphoma is the least common subtype of cHL. Only about 1% of people with cHL have this subtype. It is most common in older adults; people with the human immunodeficiency virus (HIV), the virus that causes acquired immune deficiency syndrome (AIDS); and people in non-industrialized countries. The lymph node contains almost all Reed-Sternberg cells.

Nodular lymphocyte-predominant Hodgkin lymphoma

About 5% of people with Hodgkin lymphoma have nodular lymphocyte-predominant Hodgkin lymphoma. It often develops in the lymph nodes in the neck, groin, or armpit. It is most common in younger people.

Nodular lymphocyte-predominant Hodgkin lymphoma is more similar to B-cell non-Hodgkin lymphoma. People with this type of Hodgkin lymphoma have large cells in the affected area called "popcorn cells" or "LP cells" that have a marker called CD20 on their surface. CD20 is a protein that is usually found in people diagnosed with B-cell non-Hodgkin lymphoma.

Nodular lymphocyte-predominant Hodgkin lymphoma is often treated differently from cHL. Some people with nodular lymphocyte-predominant Hodgkin lymphoma do not need treatment right away, while others may benefit from a treatment plan that includes radiation therapy, chemotherapy, or a monoclonal antibody called rituximab (Rituxan). This is explained further in Types of Treatment.

People with nodular lymphocyte-predominant Hodgkin lymphoma tend to have a very good prognosis. This means the treatment, if needed, has a very good chance of being successful and helps the patient recover. However, a small number of people with nodular lymphocyte-predominant Hodgkin lymphoma may develop a more aggressive type of non-Hodgkin lymphoma called diffuse large B-cell lymphoma through a process called transformation.

Symptoms

Hodgkin lymphoma begins subtly and symptoms develop slowly in most cases, i.e. within weeks or months. First sign of the disease is usually a painless swelling of one or more lymph nodes in the regions of the neck, clavicles, armpits and/or groins.

However, the disease can also arise from lymph nodes that can not be seen or palpated at all, such as those behind the breastbone, in the chest, abdomen or along the spine. Since the cancer is continuously growing, the affected lymph nodes will soon become occupying surrounding space, thereby impairing inner organs and their functions. Therefore, enlarged lymph nodes in certain parts of the chest (mediastinum) may cause a dry cough or breathing difficulties, while others, in the abdomen for example, can result in diffuse abdominal pain and indigestion.

Enlargement of the spleen and liver (splenomegaly, hepatomegaly) due to lymphoma cell invasion is less frequent. If the lymphocytes in the bone marrow are involved, they occupy space within the hollow interior of bones. As a result, Hodgkin lymphoma can cause reduced production of red and white blood cells and, thus, anaemia and a predisposition for infections. However, these cases are rare.

Nonspecific (general) symptoms may include fever, weight loss, drenching night sweats, fatigue, and itchy skin. The first three symptoms are frequent in patients with Hodgkin lymphoma. They are called B-symptoms.

The following overview summarizes the most frequent symptoms caused by Hodgkin lymphoma.

General symptoms

- Fever of unknown origin (over 100.4°F for three consecutive days) [B-symptom]
- Night sweats [B-symptom]
- Unexplained weight loss (more than 10 % in six consecutive months prior to admission) [B-symptom]
- Fatigue, loss of appetite, malaise
- Itchy skin

Specific symptoms

In more than 90 % of patients: painless, palpable, superficial lymph node swellings, for example in the area of the neck (most frequent location), in the armpit, above the clavicle, in the groins or simultaneously at multiple sites

- Chronic cough, shortness of breath (if thoracic lymph nodes, lungs or pleura are involved)
- Abdominal pain, back pain, diarrhea (if abdominal lymph nodes or organs, such as liver or spleen, are involved)

- Pallor due to lack of red blood cells (anaemia; if the bone marrow is involved)
- Bone or joint pain (if bones are involved)

Symptoms and complaints usually develop slowly in patients with Hodgkin lymphoma (over weeks or months). They can vary individually as to which symptoms prevail and how pronounced they are.

The occurence of one or more of the above-mentioned symptoms does not necessarily mean that they are caused by a Hodgkin lymphoma. Several of these symptoms, such as lymph node swelling and fever, are exactly those often seen with common childhood diseases like common colds and other viral infections. Nevertheless, it is strongly recommended to have the child or teenager see a paediatrician, in particular, if symptoms persist or progress.

Diagnosis

Doctors use many tests to find, or diagnose, cancer. They also do tests to learn if cancer has spread to another part of the body from where it started. If this happens, it is called metastasis. For example, imaging tests can show if the cancer has spread. Imaging tests show pictures of the inside of the body. Doctors may also do tests to learn which treatments could work best.

For most types of cancer, a biopsy is the only sure way for the doctor to know if an area of the body has cancer. In a biopsy, the doctor takes a small sample of tissue for testing in a laboratory. If a biopsy is not possible, the doctor may suggest other tests that will help make a diagnosis.

This section describes options for diagnosing this type of cancer. Your doctor may consider these factors when choosing a diagnostic test:

- The type of cancer suspected

- Your signs and symptoms

- Your age and general health

- The results of earlier medical tests

The following tests may be used to help diagnose Hodgkin lymphoma. Not all tests listed below will be used for every person.

Medical history and physical examination - The doctor will ask detailed questions about your medical history and do a physical examination, which can identify typical symptoms of Hodgkin lymphoma, such as night sweats, fevers, and enlarged lymph nodes or spleen.

Biopsy - A biopsy is the removal of a small amount of tissue for examination under a microscope. Other tests can suggest that cancer is present, but Hodgkin lymphoma can only be diagnosed after a biopsy of an affected tissue, preferably by removal (or excision) of a lymph node. Most commonly, this will be an affected lymph node in the neck, under the arm, or in the groin. If there are no lymph nodes in these areas, a biopsy of other lymph nodes, such as those in the center of the chest, may be necessary. This type of biopsy usually requires minor surgery using a procedure called mediastinoscopy. A thin, lighted tube with a camera and a cutting tool on the end is inserted into the chest through a small cut made just above the breastbone. It may also be possible to do a biopsy using a core needle. Doctors most commonly use ultrasound or a computed tomography (CT or CAT) scan to help guide the needle to the correct location.

A pathologist then analyzes the tissue sample(s) removed during the biopsy. A pathologist is a doctor who specializes in interpreting laboratory tests and evaluating cells, tissues, and organs to diagnose disease. A hematopathologist is a doctor who has received additional training in blood diseases and blood cancer diagnosis.

It is important that the biopsy sample is large enough to allow the pathologist to make an accurate diagnosis and determine the subtype of Hodgkin lymphoma. If the first biopsy does not have enough tissue to diagnose lymphoma, a second larger biopsy may be needed. As described in the Introduction, a biopsy of cHL usually has Reed-Sternberg cells. For people with nodular lymphocyte-predominant Hodgkin lymphoma, the Reed-Sternberg cells often look different and are called "LP" cells. In contrast to classic Reed-Sternberg cells, LP cancer cells have a protein on their surface called CD20.

Once Hodgkin lymphoma is diagnosed, other tests can help find out the extent of the disease, the stage, and other information to help the doctors plan treatment. These tests include:

Laboratory tests - Blood tests may include a complete blood count (CBC) and an analysis of the different types of white blood cells, in addition to the erythrocyte sedimentation rate (ESR) and liver and kidney function tests. Blood tests alone cannot detect Hodgkin lymphoma.

Computed tomography (CT or CAT) scan

A CT scan takes pictures of the inside of the body using x-rays taken from different angles. A computer combines these pictures into a detailed, 3-dimensional image that shows any abnormalities, such as enlarged lymph nodes, or tumors. A CT scan of the chest, abdomen, and pelvis can help find cancer that has spread to other parts of the body. A special dye called a contrast medium is usually given before the scan to improve the details of the images. This dye can be injected into a patient's vein or given as a pill or liquid to swallow. People with a history of kidney disease or poor kidney function should not receive a contrast medium given into a vein (intravenously or IV).

Positron emission tomography (PET) or PET-CT scan - A PET scan is usually combined with a CT scan, called a PET-CT scan. However, you may hear your doctor refer to this procedure just as a PET scan. A PET scan is a way to create pictures of organs and tissues inside the body. A small amount of a radioactive sugar substance is injected into the patient's vein. This sugar substance is taken up by cells that use the most energy. Because cancer tends to use energy actively, it absorbs more of the radioactive substance. A scanner then detects this substance to produce images of the inside of the body. PET-CT scans may be used to determine the stage of Hodgkin lymphoma. PET-CT scans may also be used to see how the lymphoma is responding to treatment.

Magnetic resonance imaging (MRI) - An MRI uses magnetic fields, not x-rays, to produce detailed images of the body. A special dye called a contrast medium is given before the scan to create a clearer picture. This dye can be injected into a patient's vein. This test is sometimes used for Hodgkin lymphoma.

Lung function tests - Also called pulmonary function tests or PFTs, lung function tests evaluate how much air the lungs can hold, how quickly air can move in and out of the lungs, and how well the lungs add oxygen and remove carbon dioxide from the blood. These tests may be done if a person's treatment plan includes chemotherapy with certain drugs that could affect the lungs.

Heart evaluation - A heart evaluation, including an echocardiogram (ECHO) or a multigated acquisition (MUGA) scan, may be used to check the function of the heart if specific types of chemotherapy will be included in a person's treatment plan.

Bone marrow aspiration and biopsy - These 2 procedures are similar and often done at the same time to examine the bone marrow. Bone marrow is the soft, spongy tissue found inside the center of bones. It has both a solid and a liquid part. A bone marrow aspiration removes a sample of the fluid with a needle. A bone marrow biopsy is the removal of a small amount of solid tissue using a needle. A pathologist then analyzes the sample. These bone marrow procedures have been mostly replaced with PET-CT scans, but they may still be done in certain situations.

After diagnostic tests are done, your doctor will review all of the results with you. If the diagnosis is Hodgkin lymphoma, these results also help the doctor describe the extent of cancer. This is called staging.

Stages

Staging helps to describe where the Hodgkin lymphoma is located, if or where it has spread, and whether it is affecting other parts of the body.

Doctors use diagnostic tests to find out the cancer's stage, so staging may not be complete until all tests are finished. Knowing the stage helps the doctor to decide what kind of treatment is best and can help predict a patient's prognosis, which is the chance of recovery. There are different stage descriptions for different types of cancer.

When staging Hodgkin lymphoma, doctors evaluate the following:

The number of cancerous lymph node areas.

Whether the cancerous lymph nodes are localized or generalized. Localized means they are located only in 1 area of the body. Generalized means they are in many areas of the body.

Whether the cancerous lymph nodes are on 1 or both sides of the diaphragm, the thin muscle under the lungs and heart that separates the chest from the abdomen.

Whether the disease has spread to the bone marrow, spleen, or extra-lymphatic organs (organs outside the lymphatic system; noted using an "E" below), such as the liver, lungs, or bone.

Lymphoma stage groupings

The stage of lymphoma describes the extent of the spread of the tumor, using the terms "stage I" to "stage IV" (1 through 4). As explained in Symptoms and Signs, each stage may also be further divided into "A" and "B" categories, based on whether or not the person is experiencing specific symptoms.

Stage I: The cancer is found in 1 lymph node region. Or, the cancer has invaded 1 extralymphatic organ or site (identified using the letter "E") but not any lymph node regions (stage IE); this is rare in Hodgkin lymphoma.

Stage II: Any of the following conditions applies:

Stage II: The cancer is in 2 or more lymph node regions on the same side of the diaphragm.

Stage IIE: The cancer involves 1 organ and its regional lymph nodes (lymph nodes located near the site of the lymphoma), with or without cancer in other lymph node regions on the same side of the diaphragm.

Stage II bulky: Either stage II or stage IIE applies, plus there is a mass in the chest. The mass is either larger than one-third the diameter of the chest or larger than 10 centimeters (cm). A centimeter is roughly equal to the width of a standard pen or pencil.

Stage III: There is cancer in lymph node areas on both sides of the diaphragm, meaning above and below it.

Stage IV: The lymphoma has spread to 1 or more organs beyond the lymph nodes. Hodgkin lymphoma usually spreads to the liver, bone marrow, or lungs.

Recurrent: Recurrent lymphoma is lymphoma that has come back after treatment. Lymphoma may return in the area where it first started or in another part of the body. Recurrence may occur at any time, including shortly after the first treatment or years later. If the lymphoma does return, there will be another round of tests to learn about the extent of the recurrence. These tests and scans are often similar to those done at the time of the original diagnosis.

Prognostic factors

In addition to stage, doctors use other prognostic factors to help plan the best treatment and predict how well this treatment will work. For people with Hodgkin lymphoma, several factors can predict whether the disease will return and which treatments will be successful. The lymphoma may be described as "high-risk disease" or "low-risk disease" based on how many of the following prognostic factors there are.

Factors that are considered less favorable and lead to a poorer prognosis include:

- Being male.
- Age 45 and older.
- Low blood albumin (a type of protein) levels, defined as less than 4 g/L.
- Low hemoglobin (red blood cell count), defined as less than 10.5 g/dL.
- White blood cell count that is more than 15,000 per cubic millimeter (mm^3).
- Lymphocyte count that is less than 600 per mm^3, less than 8% of the total white blood cell count, or both.
- Stage IV disease.

Other prognostic factors that are considered, especially for early-stage Hodgkin lymphoma, include:

- A higher erythrocyte sedimentation rate, or ESR, is associated with a poorer prognosis.
- People with lymphocyte-predominant Hodgkin lymphoma, nodular sclerosis Hodgkin lymphoma, and lymphocyte-rich classic Hodgkin lymphoma have a better prognosis, compared with other types of Hodgkin lymphoma.
- A mediastinal lymph node mass, located in the center of the chest, that is larger than 10 cm is associated with a poorer prognosis. Small mediastinal masses are not associated with a poorer prognosis.
- Having a high number of involved lymph node sites is associated with a poorer prognosis.

Treatment of HL

Hodgkin lymphoma is a type of blood cancer that involves the lymphatic system. Treatment for Hodgkin lymphoma is usually based on the stage of the condition. In some instances, a person's age, overall health, the location of the lymphoma, and other factors play a role in the type of treatment that is most effective. Because some Hodgkin treatment modalities can result in serious side effects that show up much later down the road, physicians may opt for a treatment plan with the lowest incidence of side effects.

The two primary types of treatment for Hodgkin lymphoma include chemotherapy (medications that treat cancer) and radiation therapy. In many instances, both chemotherapy and radiation are used. Other, less common forms of treatment include immunotherapy and stem cell transplant (often used when chemotherapy and radiation therapy are ineffective).

Surgery is rarely recommended to treat Hodgkin lymphoma, except when doing a biopsy (taking a small amount of tissue to test to find out if it's cancerous) and when staging (surgical removal of one or more lymph nodes to discover if the lymphoma is confined to one area, or if it has spread).

Chemotherapy

Chemotherapy is the primary treatment for those with Hodgkin lymphoma. ☐ The definition of chemotherapy (chemo) is the use of medications with the aim of killing cancer cells.

First-line chemotherapy

Newly diagnosed Hodgkin lymphoma is often treated with regimens that use a combination of chemotherapy drugs given at 1 time. The most commonly used combination of drugs in the

United States is referred to as ABVD. Another combination of drugs, known as BEACOPP, is commonly used in Europe to treat advanced Hodgkin lymphoma and is sometimes used in the United States. The drugs that make up these 2 common combinations of chemotherapy are listed below. There are other combinations that are less commonly used; not all combinations are listed here.

ABVD: Doxorubicin, bleomycin, vinblastine (Velban), and dacarbazine. ABVD chemotherapy is usually given every 2 weeks for 2 to 8 months.

AAVD: This regimen is similar to ABVD, but brentuximab vedotin (Adcetris) replaces bleomycin. AAVD is given every 2 weeks for 6 months.

BEACOPP: Bleomycin, etoposide (available as a generic drug), doxorubicin, cyclophosphamide (available as a generic drug), vincristine (Vincasar PFS), procarbazine (Matulane), and prednisone (multiple brand names). There are several different treatment schedules, but different drugs are usually given every 2 to 3 weeks.

Brentuximab vedotin (Adcetris): Brentuximab vedotin is an antibody drug conjugate. This means it delivers chemotherapy only to cells that have a special protein on the surface called CD30. The U.S. Food and Drug Administration (FDA) approved brentuximab vedotin combined with doxorubicin, vinblastine, and dacarbazine as a first-line treatment for stage III or IV cHL.

Gemcitabine combined with other drugs: Patients older than 65 to 70 years can have trouble taking a regimen of ABVD and especially BEACOPP because of the side effects. If this happens, recent research suggests that gemcitabine (Gemzar) combined with other drugs may be a good alternative.

The type of chemotherapy, number of cycles of chemotherapy, and the additional use of radiation therapy are based on the stage of the Hodgkin lymphoma and the type and number of prognostic factors. Talk with your doctor about the specifics of your treatment plan. Usually, doctors choose to monitor how well these treatments are working with repeat PET-CT scans after 2 to 3 months of treatment. If the PET scans show that the treatment is not working, the chemotherapy may be changed. If the PET scans show that treatment is working, then the doctor may decide to lower the subsequent number of drugs used or the total number of treatment cycles.

Second-line chemotherapy

There are several second-line treatments available for Hodgkin lymphoma. These are used if the lymphoma does not go into complete remission with the first treatment or if it comes back after first-line treatment with ABVD or BEACOPP, also known as a recurrence. The goals of second-line treatment may be to control the disease and its symptoms, but in many cases, they are given in preparation for an autologous stem cell transplant with the intent to achieve complete remission and cure.

ICE: Ifosfamide (Ifex), carboplatin, and etoposide. ICE is usually given every 2 or 3 weeks for 2 to 3 cycles.

ESHAP or DHAP: ESHAP is etoposide, methylprednisolone (Solu-Medrol), high-dose cytarabine, and cisplatin. DHAP is dexamethasone, high-dose cytarabine, and cisplatin. ESHAP or DHAP regimens are given every 3 weeks for 2 to 3 cycles.

GVD, Gem-Ox, or GDP: GVD is gemcitabine, vinorelbine (Navelbine), and doxorubicin. Gem-Ox is gemcitabine and oxaliplatin (Eloxatin). GDP is gemcitabine, dexamethasone, and cisplatin. Gemcitabine-based regimens are either given 2 weeks in a row followed by an off-week or every other week.

Brentuximab vedotin: This drug is an important treatment option if previous chemotherapy stops working. Brentuximab vedotin is usually given every 3 weeks for up to 16 cycles, although sometimes it is given every 4 weeks. It is being tested as an adjunct or replacement for chemotherapy before stem cell transplantation in people with recurrent Hodgkin lymphoma. It was also approved in 2015 by the FDA for use in certain people after stem cell transplantation who are at a high risk for recurrence.

Bendamustine (Treanda): Bendamustine is generally given every 4 weeks. Sometimes it is combined with other drugs listed above to treat Hodgkin lymphoma that has come back after treatment.

It is unclear which of these chemotherapy treatments is best for people with Hodgkin lymphoma. The best treatment may differ depending on the type and stage of the lymphoma. For this reason, many clinical trials are being done to compare these different treatments. These clinical trials are designed to find out which combination works best with the fewest short-term and long-term side effects.

During chemotherapy, your doctors will usually repeat some of the original tests, especially PET-CT scans. These tests are used to watch the lymphoma and see how well treatment is working.

The side effects of chemotherapy depend on the individual and the doses used, but they can include fatigue, risk of infection, nausea and vomiting, peripheral neuropathy (tingling or pain in the fingers and toes), hair loss, loss of appetite, and constipation. These side effects usually go away after treatment is finished. Although the risk of long-term side effects has decreased as treatments have improved, chemotherapy still can cause long-term side effects. These late effects, which can develop 10 or more years after treatment ends, may include second cancers, especially among those who were treated with radiation therapy, and diseases of the heart or blood vessels. People with lymphoma may also have concerns about if or how their treatment may affect their sexual health and fertility. Talk about these topics with the health care team before treatment begins. Learn more about late effects of treatment.

Immunotherapy

Immunotherapy is a type of drug therapy to help the body's immune system recognize and destroy cancer cells more effectively.

Monoclonal Antibodies

The body makes proteins called antibodies to help fight infections. Monoclonal antibodies can be synthetically made to attack specific targets. The target differs depending on the type of cancer. Monoclonal antibodies attack cancer cells, but not the cells that are healthy. Examples of drugs in this classification that treat Hodgkin lymphoma include:

- Rituxan (rituximab)
- Adcetris (brentuximab vedotin)

For people with a high risk of recurrence of Hodgkin's disease, brentuximab may be given for a year after stem cell transplant. It is administered intravenously, commonly ordered every three weeks.

Common side effects of brentuximab include:

- Fatigue
- Nausea and Vomiting
- Diarrhea
- Fever
- Infections
- Low blood cell counts

- Neuropathy (damage to nerves)

More Common side effects of rituximab may include: □

- Fatigue
- Headache
- Fever and chills
- Nausea
- Rash
- Increase the risk of infection for several months after the drug has been discontinued

More severe side effects could occur during the infusion of any type of monoclonal antibodies, but this is rare. The physician will administer medication that helps to prevent severe reactions. If a reaction does occur during the initial infusion, it's rare that it will recur with subsequent doses.

The drug rituximab may cause hepatitis B infections to recur. This could lead to liver problems or even death. It's important to tell your health care providers if you have had hepatitis B in the past before starting on rituximab.

Radiation

Radiation therapy is used to kill cancer cells with the use of high-energy rays. This type of treatment is considered the most beneficial when Hodgkin lymphoma affects only one area of the body.

Radiation treatments are given much like an X-ray is taken, but the radiation is much stronger than that of an X-ray. Radiation therapy is painless and takes only a few minutes, but the preparation for the treatment may take longer. Special shields are used to prevent radiation from targeting healthy, surrounding tissue; young children may need to be sedated so they will stay still during the treatment.

Side Effects

Due to the long-term side effects of radiation therapy, it's usually given in low doses.

Short-term side effects may include:

- Redness, blistering or peeling of skin in the area where treatment is administered
- Dry mouth
- Fatigue
- Diarrhea
- Nausea
- Low blood counts and increased risk of infection (when radiation is administered in several areas of the body)

Long-term side effects may include:

- Damage to the thyroid gland (if radiation is administered in the neck area)
- Abnormal bone growth (in children) which could result in deformities
- An increased risk of heart attacks and stroke
- An increased risk of other types of cancer

Stem Cell Transplants

Stem cell transplants may be used to treat Hodgkin lymphoma that does not respond completely to chemotherapy. High doses of chemotherapy may then be used to kill the cancerous cells, but this also damages the ability of the bone marrow to produce blood cells. Stem cell transplants replenish the body's ability to produce normal blood cells after high doses of chemotherapy are given.

There are two primary methods of stem cell transplantation; from different sources of stem cells.

An autologous stem cell transplant uses stem cells collected from a person's own blood, which is harvested before the transplant procedure. While the person is getting chemo, radiation treatment, or both, the stem cells are frozen, then thawed once Hodgkin treatment is complete. Once the person is ready to receive the procedure, the stem cells are administered intravenously. For Hodgkin lymphoma, an autologous stem cell transplant is the most common type of transplant.

The second type of transplant is an allogeneic stem cell transplant, in which the stem cells come from a donor.

Alternative cancer treatments

We are fighting with cancer since the dawn of history. Every year we discover new diagnostic modalities, better radiotherapy techniques and lots of new chemotherapy drugs. But we have completely failed to defeat this disease called cancer. Think again, are we really going on the right path? Does conventional Medicine really targets upon the prime cause of cancer?

It's not that more effective alternative treatments for cancer don't exist – they most certainly do. It's just that the allopathic system isn't at all interested in divulging real cures. This is because their expensive therapies generate billions of dollars for the cancer industry.

Chemotherapy Doesn't Cure Cancer – It Causes It!

Chemotherapy does, in fact, kill cancer cells. But it also kills healthy cells, along with a patient's immune system and, really, anything else that crosses its path. At worst, such treatments kill patients more quickly than if they had chosen not to undergo them at all.

There's no money to be made in prescribing prevention advice like eating fewer chemicals and exercising more. The "bread and butter" of the cancer industry is unleashing the next, latest-and-greatest cancer drug. Not telling you how to avoid cancer in the first place.

Many people with cancer are interested in trying any treatment that may cure them safely, including complementary and alternative cancer treatments. There is growing evidence that these alternative cancer treatments give wonderful results. Here are some alternative cancer treatments that are very safe and effective.

Budwig Protocol - The best Alternative Treatment effective in all cancers and all stages with documented 90% success

Laetrile (Vitamin B-17) Therapy
Gerson Therapy
Dr. Simoncini Baking Soda Cancer Treatment
High-dose vitamin C
Frankincense Essential Oil Therapy
Immunotherapy
Hyperthermia
Oxygen Therapy and Hyperbaric Chambers

Laetrile (Vitamin B-17) Therapy

Introduction

During 1950, after many years of research, a dedicated biochemist Dr. Ernest T. Krebs Jr., isolated a new vitamin from bitter apricot kernel that he called 'B-17' or 'Laetrile'. He conducted further lab animal and culture experiments to conclude that laetrile would be effective in the treatment of cancer. As the years rolled by, thousands became convinced that Krebs had finally found the treatment for all cancers. He proposed that cancer was caused by a deficiency of Vitamin B 17 (Laetrile, Amygdaline).

To prove that it was not toxic to humans he injected it into his own arm. As he predicted, there were no harmful or distressing side effects. The Laetrile had no harmful effect on normal cells but was deadly to cancer cells. Dr. Ernst Krebs stated that we need at least a minimum of 100 mg of B-17 or around 7 bitter apricot seeds to almost guarantee a cancer free life.

Nitriloside is a beta-cyanophoric glycosides, a large group of water-soluble, sugar-containing compounds found in a number of plants. Amygdalin is one of the most common nitrilosides. Laetrile is a partly man-made molecule and shares only part of the Amygdalin structure. Both Laetrile and Amygdalin have been promoted as "Vitamin B-17".

Laetrile stands for laevo-rotatory mandelonitrile beta-diglucoside. The "laevo" part references a purified form of B-17 that turns polarized light in a left-turning direction. Dr. Krebs, Jr. believed that only the left-rotating Laevo form was effective against cancer. So it's important to check the purity of your Laetrile.

How B-17 works (A tale of two enzymes)

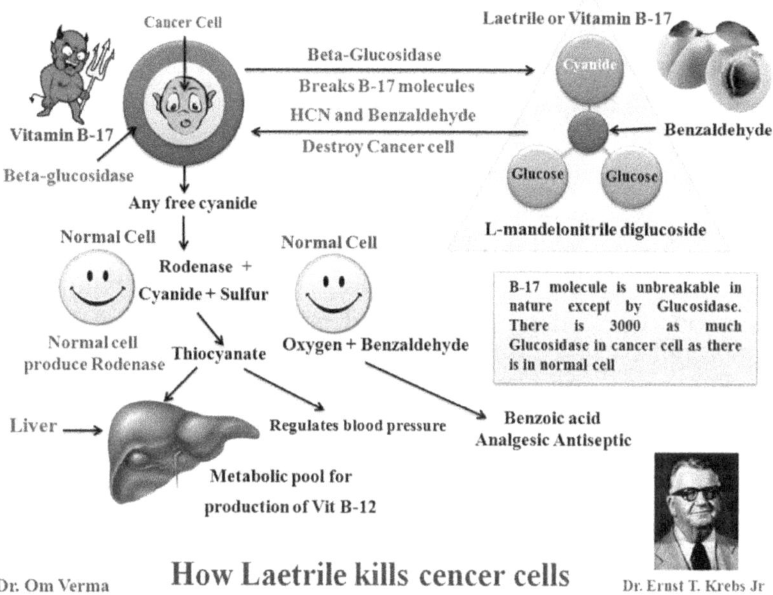

How Laetrile kills cencer cells

Laetrile, commonly known as Vitamin B-17 or Amygdalin, contains two units of Sugar, one of Benzaldehyde and one of Cyanide, all tightly locked within it. Everyone knows that cyanide can be highly toxic and even fatal if taken in sufficient quantity. However, as it is in locked state is completely inert and absolutely has no effect on living tissue. There is only one substance that can unlock this molecule and release the cyanide. That substance is an enzyme called beta-glucocidase, which we shall call the unlocking enzyme. When B-17 comes in contact with this enzyme, not only the cyanide is released but also Benzaldehyde which is highly toxic by itself. In fact, these two working together are at least 100 times more poisonous to cancer cell than either of them separately. The unlocking enzyme is not

113

found to any dangerous degree anywhere in the body except at the cancer cell where it is present in great quantity. The result is that Vit B-17 is unlocked at the cancer cells becomes poisonous to the cancer cells and only to the cancer cells.

There is another important enzyme called Rodanese, which we shall identify as protecting enzyme. The reason is that it has the ability to neutralize cyanide by converting it instantly into the byproducts (thiocyanate) that actually are beneficial and essential for health. This enzyme is found in great quantities in every part of the body except the cancer cells which consequently is not protected. Here then is a biochemical process that destroys cancer cells while at the same time nourishing and sustaining non-cancerous cells. It is intricate and perfect mechanism of nature that simply couldn't be accidental.

Laetrile - Metabolic Therapy

Metabolic therapy is a non-toxic cancer treatment based on the use of Vitamin B- 17, proteolytic pancreatic enzymes, immuno-stimulants, and vitamin and mineral supplements.

There are three parts to this program:

Laetrile

Vitamins and enzymes

Diet

Phase I Metabolic - Program for the first 21 days

Laetrile

Amygdalin (Laetrile) is available in 500 mg. tablets and in vials (10 cc 3 Gm) for intravenous use. Both forms are used. Two vials of Laetrile are given IV three times weekly for three weeks with at least one day between injections (Mon., Wed., Fri.). Dose of Amygdalin Tablets 500 mg is 2 tab three times a day with meals on the days on which the patients do not receive the intravenous Laetrile. Thiocyanate levels in the blood can be measured during treatment. In general, the patients who do best are those in whom the thiocyanate level is between 1.2 and 2.5 Mg/DL (Philip E.Binzel   ).

Vitamins and Enzymes

Preven-Ca Caps - Preven-Ca is a comprehensive blend of potent herb and fruit extracts, designed to provide a broad Spectrum of Flavonoids with scientifically demonstrated Antioxidant activity and effectiveness. One capsule with each meal.

Vitamin B15 - One capsule three times a daily at the end of each meal.

Megazyme Forte (Proteolytic Enzymes) Three tablets two hours after each meal (9 daily).

Ester Vitamin C 1000 mg capsule - One capsule with each meal.

Shark Cartilage It has been said that Sharks are the healthiest creature on earth. Sharks are immune to practically every disease known to man. One capsules three times a daily with each meal.

Natural Vitamin E 400 iu - One gel with lunch and one with dinner.

AHCC (Active Hexose Correlated Compound) - Two capsules with each meal.

Multi Vitamin & Mineral Liquid - 1 oz (two tablespoons) once daily with a meal.

Vitamin A & E Emulsion - 5 drops in juice or water three times per day.

Barley Grass Juice - One teaspoon in juice three times per day.

Bitter apricot seeds - No more than 12 every 2 hours 6 times a day.

Dimethyl sulfoxide (DMSO) - DMSO is a by-product of the wood and paper industry. It is known for its ability to permeate living tissue and stimulate cellular processes.

Or Phase 1 Oral

Injectable Amygdalin is replaced with 500mg Amygdalin tablets. Binzel recommends 2 of these tablets with each meal for a total of 6 per day. Otherwise the ORAL Phase 1 includes the same materials as above.

Phase 2 Metabolic - Program for the next 3 months

It comprises the same materials as Phase 1 except that the dosages for the vitamin B-17 as well as the A&E Emulsion Drops change to the following:

Vitamin B-17 500 mg tablets: 1 tablet with each meal and one at bedtime.

Vitamin A & E emulsion drops: 10 drops in juice or water two times per day (suspend for 2 months after 3 months of use).

Diet

Consume those fruits (i.e. seeds), grains and nuts that are rich in laetrile. Consume salads with healthy dressings. For protein patient should consume whole grains including corn, beans, buckwheat, nuts, dried fruits. Real butter in small amounts is permitted. The patients are not permitted anything which contains white flour or white sugar. Take away all meat, all poultry, all fish, all eggs and milk from patients. Margarine is detrimental to good nutrition. No coffee is permitted.

Zinc acts as transport vehicle for laetrile in the body. If patient does not have sufficient zinc, laetrile will not get into the tissues of the body. That's why you should give a spoonful of pumpkin seeds along with bitter apricot kernels. The body will not rebuild any tissue without sufficient quantities of Vitamin C etc.

The Gerson Therapy

The Gerson Therapy is a natural treatment that activates the body's extraordinary ability to heal itself through an organic, plant-based diet, raw juices, coffee enemas and natural supplements.

With its whole-body approach to healing, the Gerson Therapy naturally reactivates your body's magnificent ability to heal itself – with no damaging side effects. This a powerful, natural treatment boosts the body's own immune system to heal cancer, arthritis, heart disease, allergies, and many other degenerative diseases. Dr. Max Gerson developed the Gerson Therapy in the 1930s, initially as a treatment for his own debilitating migraines, and eventually as a treatment for degenerative diseases such as skin tuberculosis, diabetes and, most famously, cancer.

An abundance of nutrients from copious amounts of fresh, organic juices are consumed every day, providing your body with a super-dose of enzymes, minerals and nutrients. These substances then break down diseased tissue in the body, while coffee enemas aid in eliminating toxins from the liver.

Throughout our lives our bodies are being filled with a variety of carcinogens and toxic pollutants. These toxins reach us through the air we breathe, the food we eat, the medicines we take and the water we drink. The Gerson Therapy's intensive detoxification regimen eliminates these toxins from the body, so that true healing can begin.

How the Gerson Therapy Works

The Gerson Therapy regenerates the body to health, supporting each important metabolic requirement by flooding the body with nutrients from about 15- 20 pounds of organically-grown fruits and vegetables daily. Most is used to make fresh raw juice, up to one glass every hour, up to 13 times per day. Raw and cooked solid foods are generously consumed. Oxygenation is usually more than doubled, as oxygen deficiency in the blood contributes to many degenerative diseases. The metabolism is also stimulated through the addition of thyroid, potassium and other supplements, and by avoiding heavy animal fats, excess protein, sodium and other toxins.

Degenerative diseases render the body increasingly unable to excrete waste materials adequately, commonly resulting in liver and kidney failure. The Gerson Therapy uses intensive detoxification to eliminate wastes, regenerate the liver, reactivate the immune system and restore the body's essential defenses – enzyme, mineral and hormone systems. With generous, high-quality nutrition, increased oxygen availability, detoxification, and improved metabolism, the cells – and the body – can regenerate, become healthy and prevent future illness.

Juicing

Fresh-pressed juice from raw foods provides the easiest and most effective way of providing high-quality nutrition. By juicing, patients can take in the nutrients and enzymes from nearly 15 pounds of produce every day, in a manner that is easy to digest and absorb.

Every day, a typical patient on the Gerson Therapy for cancer consumes up to thirteen glasses of fresh, raw carrot-apple and green leaf juices. These juices are prepared hourly from fresh, raw, organic fruits and vegetables, using a two-step juicer or a masticating juicer used with a separate hydraulic press.

The Gerson Therapy Diet

The Gerson Therapy diet is plant-based and entirely organic. The diet is naturally high in vitamins, minerals, enzymes, micro-nutrients, and extremely low in sodium, fats, and proteins. The following is a typical daily diet for a Gerson patient on the full therapy regimen:

> Thirteen glasses of fresh, raw carrot-apple and green-leaf juices prepared hourly from fresh, organic fruits and vegetables.
>
> Three full plant-based meals, freshly prepared from organically grown fruits, vegetables and whole grains. A typical meal will include salad, cooked vegetables, baked potatoes, Hippocrates soup and juice.
>
> Fresh fruit and vegetables available at all hours for snacking, in addition to the regular diet.

Supplements

All medications used in connection with the Gerson Therapy are classed as biologicals, materials of organic origin that are supplied in therapeutic amounts. The supplements used on the Gerson Therapy include:

> Potassium compound
> Lugol's solution
> Vitamin B-12
> Thyroid hormone
> Pancreatic Enzymes

Detoxification

Coffee enemas are the primary method of detoxification of the tissues and blood on the Gerson Therapy. Coffee enemas accomplish this essential task, assisting the liver in eliminating toxic residues from the body for good. Cancer patients on the Gerson Therapy may take up to 5 coffee enemas per day. The Gerson Therapy also utilizes castor oil to stimulate bile flow and enhance the liver's ability to filter blood.

Simoncini's Baking Soda Cancer Treatment

Dr. Tullio Simoncini is a medical doctor in Italy who has done more than anyone to explore the uses of the baking soda cancer treatment as an alternative cancer treatment. It is known that cancer creates and favors an acid environment and because of this, Dr. Simoncini and others have used sodium bicarbonate as an alkaline therapeutic agent.

The way that acidity seems to protect cancer is not fully understood. It seems that cytotoxic T-cells, which may attack cancer cells under normal conditions, are inactivated in an acid extracellular fluid. Also, the type of acidity that cancer produces, i.e., lactic acid, stimulates vascular endothelial growth factor and angiogenesis. This is like a highway project, which enables a tumor to build the blood vessels that it needs to bring the nutrients for it to survive. So the tumor creates an environment in which it can then exist comfortably.

Baking Soda's Alkalinity Fights Cancer's Acidity

At a pH of about 10, sodium bicarbonate is an antidote to this acidity. It can be used clinically in sterile, intravenous form. This is a liquid, sterile bicarbonate of soda. The baking soda cancer treatment is well-tolerated, even with frequent repeated dosing. Dr. Simonchini also injects soda bicarb solution directly into the tumors at his center.

Cancer a Fungus problem?

Dr. Simonchini says that cancer is caused by fungus However, it is useful to know that not only does sodium bicarbonate disrupt the comfortable environment of tumors, but it also has anti-fungal effect.

Best Alternative Treatment - Budwig Protocol

90% documented success in all types of Cancers

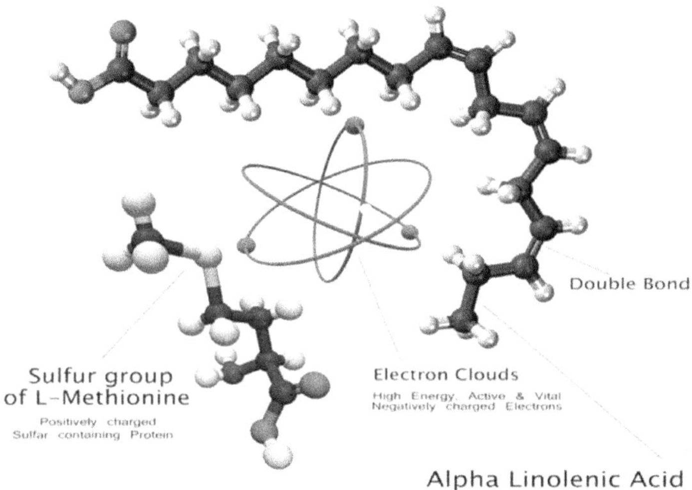

Dr. Budwig has been referred to as a top European cancer research scientist, biochemist, pharmacologist, and physicist. Dr. Budwig was a seven-time Nobel Prize nominee.

In Germany in 1952, she was the central government's senior expert for fats and pharmaceutical drugs. She's considered one of the world's leading authorities on fats and oils. Her research has shown the tremendous effects that commercially processed fats and oils (having Trans fatty acids) have in destroying cell membranes and lowering the voltage in the cells of our bodies, which then result in chronic and terminal disease including cancer.

What we have forgotten is that we are body electric. The cells of our body fire electrically. They have a nucleus in the center of the cell which is positively charged, and the cell membrane, which is the outer lining of the cell, is negatively charged. We are all aware of how fats clog up our veins and arteries and are the leading cause of heart attacks, but we never looked beyond the end of our noses to see how these very dangerous fats and oils are affecting the overall health of our minds and bodies at the cellular level.

Dr. Budwig discovered that when unsaturated fats have been chemically treated, their unsaturated qualities are destroyed and the field of electrons removed. This commercial processing of fats destroys the field of electrons that the cell membranes (60-75 trillion cells) in our bodies must have to fire properly (i.e. function properly).

The fats' ability to associate with protein and thereby to achieve water solubility in the fluids of the living body is destroyed. As Budwig put it, "the battery is dead because the electrons in these fats and oils recharge it." When the electrons are destroyed the fats are no longer active and cannot flow into the capillaries and through the fine capillary networks. This is when circulation problems arise.

Without the proper metabolism of fats in our bodies, every vital function and every organ is affected. This includes the generation of new life and new cells. Our bodies produce over 500 million new cells daily. Dr. Budwig points out that in growing new cells, there is a polarity between the electrically positive nucleus and the electrically negative cell membrane with its high unsaturated fatty acids. During cell division, the cell, and new daughter cell must contain enough electron-rich fatty acids in the cell's surface area to divide off completely from the old cell. When this process is interrupted the body begins to die. In essence, these commercially processed fats and oils are shutting down the electrical field of the cells allowing chronic and terminal diseases to take hold of our bodies.

A very good example would be tumors. Dr. Budwig noted that "The formation of tumors usually happens as follows. In those body areas which normally host many growth processes, such as in the skin and membranes, the glandular organs, for example, the liver and pancreas or the glands in the stomach and intestinal tract—it is here that the growth processes are brought to a standstill. Because the polarity is missing, due to the lack of electron rich highly unsaturated fat, the course of growth is disturbed—the surface-active fats are not present; the substance becomes inactive before the maturing and shedding process of the cells ever takes place, which results in the formation of tumors."

She pointed out that this can be reversed by providing the simple foods, cottage cheese, and flax seed oil, which revises the stagnated growth processes. This naturally causes the tumor or tumors present to dissolve and the whole range of symptoms which indicate a "dead battery are cured." Dr. Budwig did not believe in the use of growth-inhibiting treatments such as chemotherapy or radiation. She was quoted as saying "I flat declare that the usual hospital treatments today, in a case of tumorous growth, most certainly leads to worsening of the disease or a speedier death, and in healthy people, quickly causes cancer."

Dr. Budwig discovered that when she combined flaxseed oil, with its powerful healing nature of essential electron rich unsaturated fats, and cottage cheese, which is rich in sulfur protein, the bonding produced makes the oil water soluble and easily absorbed into the cell membrane.

I found testimonials of people from around the world who had been diagnosed with terminal cancer (all types of cancer), sent home to die and were now living healthy, normal lives. Not only had Dr. Budwig been using her protocol for treating cancer in Europe, but she also treated other chronic diseases such as arthritis, heart infarction, irregular heartbeat, psoriasis, eczema (other skin diseases), immune deficiency syndromes (Multiple Sclerosis and other autoimmune diseases), diabetes, lungs (respiratory conditions), stomach ulcers, liver, prostate, strokes, brain tumors, brain (strengthens activity), arteriosclerosis and other chronic diseases. Dr. Budwig's protocol proved successful where orthodox traditional medicine was failing.

Prime Cause of Cancer

We are fighting with cancer since the dawn of history. Every year we discover new diagnostic modalities, better radiotherapy techniques and lots of new chemotherapy drugs. But we have completely failed to defeat this disease called cancer. Think again, are we really going on the right path? Does conventional Medicine really targets upon the prime cause of cancer???

Otto Warburg – Biography

Otto Heinrich Warburg (October 8, 1883 – August 1, 1970), son of physicist Emil Warburg, was a German physiologist, medical doctor and Nobel laureate. His mother was the daughter of a Protestant family of bankers and civil servants from Baden. Warburg studied chemistry under the great Emil Fischer, and earned his "Doctor of Chemistry" in Berlin in 1906. He then earned the degree of "Doctor of Medicine" in Heidelberg in 1911. Between 1908 and 1914, Warburg was affiliated with the Naples Marine Biological Station, in Naples, Italy, where he conducted research.

He served as an officer in the elite Uhlan (cavalry regiment) during the First World War, and was given the Iron Cross (1st Class) award for his bravery. Warburg is considered one of the 20th century's leading biochemists. Towards the end of the war, Albert Einstein, who had been a friend of Warburg's father Emil, wrote Warburg asking him to leave the army and return to academia, since it would be a tragedy for the world to lose his talents. Einstein and Warburg later became friends, and Einstein's work in physics had great influence on Otto's biochemical research.

While working at the Marine Biological Station, Warburg performed research on oxygen consumption in sea urchin eggs after fertilization, and proved that upon fertilization, the rate of respiration increases by as much as six fold. His experiments also proved that iron is essential for the development of the larval stage.

In 1918, Warburg was appointed professor at the Kaiser Wilhelm Institute for Biology in Berlin-Dahlem. By 1931 he was promoted as director of the Kaiser Wilhelm Institute for Cell Physiology, which was later on, renamed the Max Planck Society. Warburg investigated the metabolism of tumors and the respiration of cells, particularly cancer cells, and in 1931 was awarded the Nobel Prize in Physiology for his "discovery of the nature and mode of action of the respiratory enzyme."

Nomination for a second Nobel Prize

In 1944, Warburg was nominated for a second Nobel Prize in Physiology by Albert Szent-Györgyi, for his work on nicotinamide, the mechanism and enzymes involved in fermentation, and the discovery of flavin (in yellow enzymes), but was prevented from receiving it by Adolf Hitler's regime.

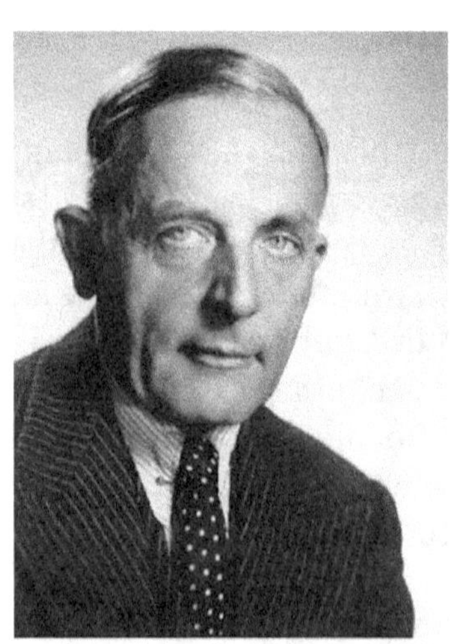
Dr. Otto Warburg (Oct 8, 1883 Aug 1, 1970)

Otto Warburg edited and had much of his original work published in The Metabolism of Tumors and wrote New Methods of Cell Physiology (1962). Otto Warburg was thrilled when Oxford University awarded him an honorary doctorate.

In his later years, Warburg was convinced that illness is resulted from pollution; this caused him to become a bit of a health advocate. He insisted on eating bread made from wheat grown organically on his farm. When he visited restaurants, he often made arrangements to pay the full price for a cup of tea, but to only be served boiling water, from which he would make tea with a tea bag he had brought with him. He was also known to go to significant lengths to obtain organic butter, the quality of which he trusted.

The Otto Warburg Medal

The Otto Warburg Medal is intended to commemorate Warburg's outstanding achievements. It has been awarded by the German Society for Biochemistry and Molecular Biology since 1963. The prize honors and encourages pioneering achievements in fundamental biochemical and molecular biological research. The Otto Warburg Medal is regarded as the highest award for biochemists and molecular biologists in Germany.

Prime cause of Cancer

Warburg hypothesized that cancer growth is caused by tumor cells mainly generating energy (as e.g. adenosine triphosphate / ATP) by anaerobic breakdown of glucose (known as fermentation, or anaerobic respiration). This is in contrast to healthy cells, which mainly generate energy from oxidative breakdown of pyruvate. Pyruvate is an end product of glycolysis, and is oxidized within the mitochondria. Hence, and according to Warburg, cancer should be interpreted as a mitochondrial dysfunction.

In short, Warburg summarized that all normal cells absolutely require oxygen, but cancer cells can live without oxygen - a rule without exception. Deprive a cell 35% of its oxygen for 48 hours and it would become cancerous. **Dr. Otto Warburg clearly mentioned that the root cause of cancer is lack of oxygen in the cells.**

He also discovered that cancer cells are anaerobic (do not breathe oxygen), get the energy by fermenting glucose and produce levo-rotating lactic acid, and the body becomes acidic. Cancer cannot survive in the presence of high levels of oxygen, as found in an alkaline state.

He postulated that sulfur containing protein and some unknown fat is required to attract oxygen into the cell. This fat plays a major role in the respiration and functioning of Warburg respiratory enzyme. He thought it would be butyric acid and made experiment, but this attempt was a failure. For many decades scientists were trying to identify this unknown and mysterious fat but nobody succeeded (Otto Warburg, Wikipedia).

Dr. Johanna Budwig - Biography & Science

Birth of an angel

A lovely couple, Hermann Budwig and Elisabeth, lived in Essen town of Germany situated on the bank of river Ruhr. On the eve of 30th September, 1908 Elisabeth delivered a brilliant and lucky angel. Hermann and 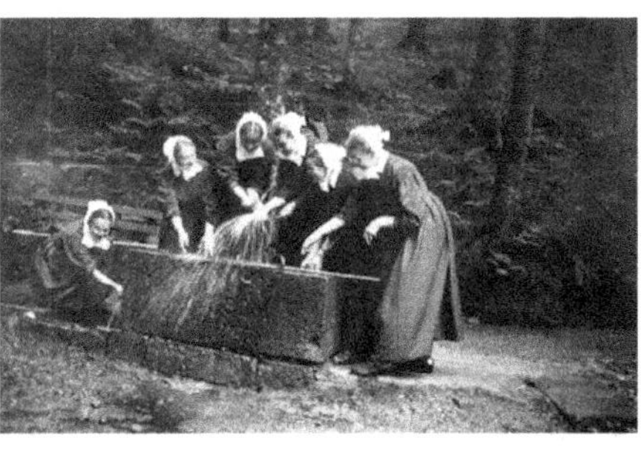 Elisabeth were very happy, and celebrating. They called her Johanna. In German, Johanna means a gift from God. In the family and neighborhood everybody was talking that Johanna is very lucky, she will study in a college and become a big doctor. Actually, 1908 was very fortunate and important year for the freedom of women in Germany. Government for the first time in history, changed laws, and allowed women to study in college and Universities. Also the German parliament passed a legislation to allow women to become members of political parties and prestigious clubs. Though women were given new rights and freedom, liberalization was slow and old values still persisted.

The tough life of a sage of science

Unluckily, Elisabeth died in 1920; family members thought that her father, being a poor loco mechanic, might not look after Johanna. So she was sent to an orphanage. This was a great shock for the little Johanna, but it had one positive side also. Education up to higher level was totally free for orphans.

In 1926, Germany was slowly recovering from the after effects of the First World War. Economic conditions were improving. Scholars and scientists were developing new technologies in every field. One third of all Nobel Prizes were being given to German academics.

Deaconess at Kaiserswerth

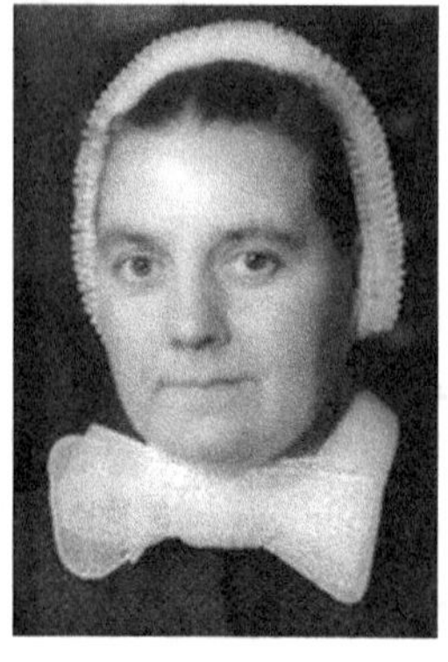

Johanna was very intelligent and sharp in studies from the beginning. In order to achieve good future, she decided to join the renowned Deaconess's Institute of Kaiserswerth in 1925. Theodor Fliedner, a pastor, founded Kaiserswerth Institute for welfare of unmarried mothers, prisoners, patients, orphans and poor children in 1836. In the beginning a Hospital and a Nursing School was established. This school was very famous Nursing School of that time. Florence Nightingale, known as mother of modern nursing, also studied in this Deaconess School in 1850. Intelligent Johanna easily got admission in this Institute. She was made a "deaconess" on March 30, 1932. This was the most appropriate place for her. There was a 1000 bedded hospital, pharmacy and a boarding school. She decided to study pharmacy.

After completing preliminary education in Kaiserswerth, she joined Münster University for further studies. Her analytical thinking and precise knowledge was noticed by her Professor Dr Hans Paul Kaufmann. He always encouraged and helped her. Here she passed state examination in pharmacy and was rewarded distinction in chemistry in 1936. Then she continued further education in physics, and received the title "Doctor of Science" at the University of Münster in 1938. On August 1, 1939, she was appointed as in-charge of pharmacy at the Military Hospital in Kaiserswerth.

Next month, Hitler's military forces attacked Poland. During war time, brave Johanna was busy in organizing and expanding the pharmacy. The war was not an easy time. There were two thousand people living in Kaiserswerth. Johanna was responsible for ensuring that there were enough medicines in this time of rationing and a thriving black market. She was well prepared and ready to fulfill any emergency demand for her patients. Many of her fellow deaconesses were often jealous and not co-operating but she continued evolving her professional skills. She was strong and was confronting every opponent (Dr. Johanna Budwig Stiftung).

Dr Budwig's scientific thinking, work and career

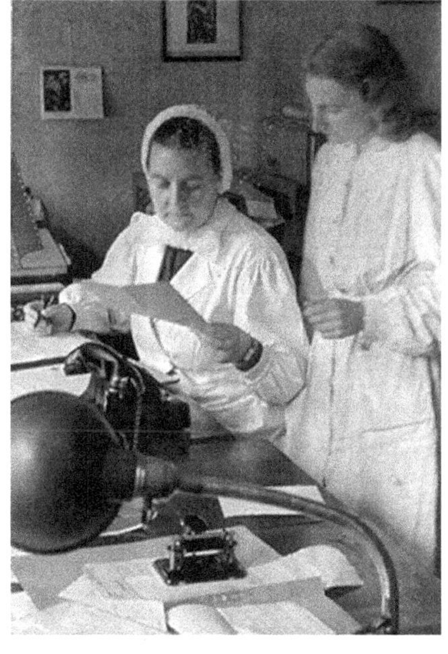

After Second World War, Johanna left Kaiserswerth in 1949. Soon Prof. Kaufmann came to know that she had left Kaiserswerth. He immediately met and persuaded her to work with him in Münster University, as he was always impressed from her talent. He converted the basement of his house into a laboratory and arranged all facilities for her research. He was famous as Fat Pope in the whole Europe.

On Prof. Kaufmann's recommendation, Johanna was appointed as the chief expert for drugs and fats at the Federal Institute for Fats Research, Germany. This was the country's largest office issuing the approval of new drugs used for cancer. Many applications had been submitted to her for approval. These were the medications for cancer therapy with the sulfhydryl group (sulfur-containing protein compounds). Everywhere she saw that fats played a role in cellular respiration, also in expert reports provided by well-known professors like Prof. Nonnenbruch. Unfortunately, fats could only be detected in the late stage, and there were no method to distinguish between fats chemically.

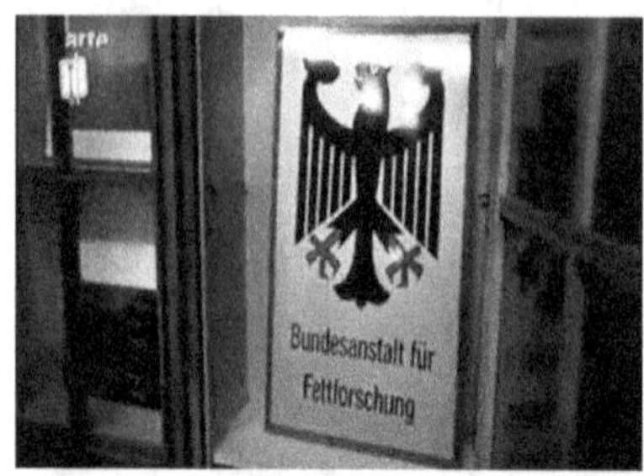

By this time, she developed paper chromatography. With this technique for first time she was able to detect fatty acids and lipoproteins directly even in 0.1 ml of blood. She used Co60 isotopes successfully to produce the first differential reaction for fatty acids, and produced the first direct iodine value via radioiodine. She also developed control of atmosphere in a closed system by using gas systems which act as antioxidants. She further developed Coloring methods, separating effects of fats and fatty acids. She too studied their behavior in blue and red light with fluorescent dyes.

Using rhodamine red dye, she studied the electrical behavior of the unsaturated fatty acids with their "halo". With this technique she could prove that electron rich highly unsaturated Linoleic and Linolenic fatty acids (Flax oil being the richest source) were the mysterious and undiscovered decisive fats required to attract oxygen into the cells, which Otto Warburg could not find. She studied the electromagnetic function of pi-electrons of the linolenic acid in the cell membranes, for nerve function, secretions,

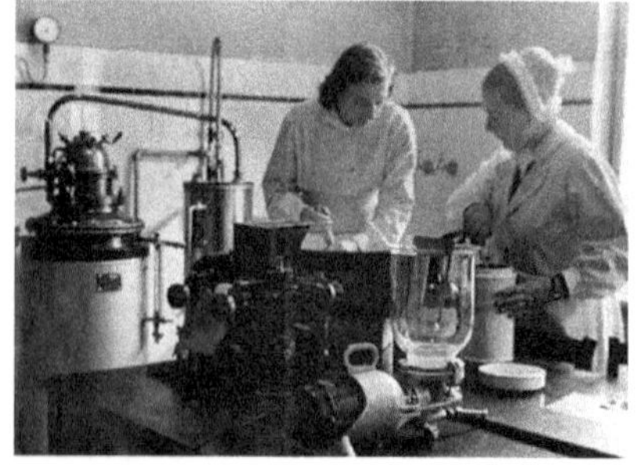

mitosis, as well as cell division. She also examined the synergism of the sulfur containing protein with the pi-electrons of the highly unsaturated fatty acids and their significance for the formation of the hydrogen bridge between fat and protein, which represent "the only path" for fast and focused Transport of electrons during respiration. This research was extensively published in 1950 in Neue Wege in der Fettforschung (New Directions in Fat Research) and other publications.

This immediately caused an excitement and turmoil in the scientific community. Everybody thought that it would open new doors in Cancer research. She also proved that hydrogenated fats and refined oils including all Trans-fatty acids were not having vital electrons and were respiratory poisons.

During her research, she found that the blood of seriously ill cancer patients had deficiency of unsaturated essential fats (Linoleic and Linolenic fatty acids), lipoproteins, phosphatides, and hemoglobin. She also had noticed that cancer 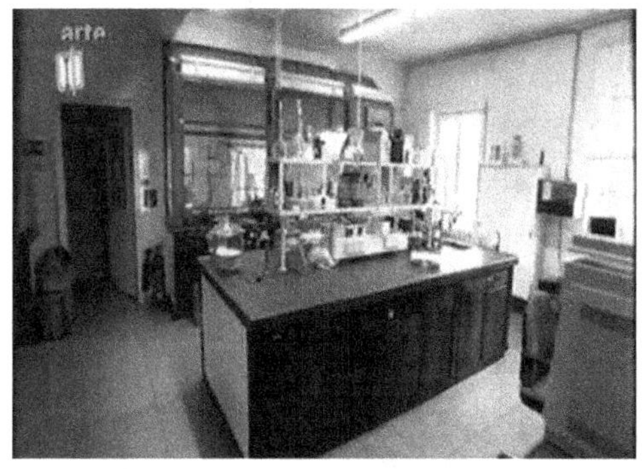 patients had a strange greenish-yellow substance in their blood which is not present in the blood of healthy people (Budwig, Cancer The Problem And The Solution).

She wanted to develop a healing program for cancer. So she enrolled over 642 cancer patients from four hospitals in Münster. She gave Flax oil and Cottage Cheeseto these patients. After just three months, patients began to improve in health and strength, the yellow green substance in their blood began to disappear, tumors gradually receded and at the same time the nutrients began to rise.

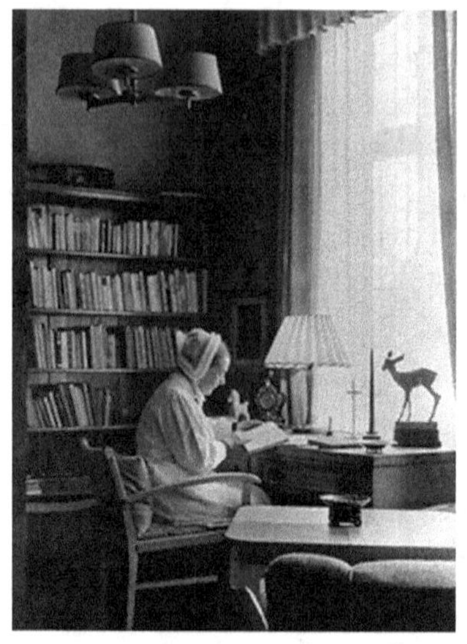

This way she developed a simple cure for cancer, based on the consumption of Flax oil with low fat Quark or cottage cheese, raw organic diet, mild exercise, Flax oil massage and the healing powers of the sun. It was a great victory and the first milestone in the battle against cancer. She treated approx. 2500 cancer patients during last few decades. Prof. Halme of surgery clinic in Helsinki used to keep records of her patients. According to him her success was over 90%, and this was achieved in cases, which were rejected by Allopathic doctors.

Dr. Budwig was a courageous scientist. She **loudly and convincingly argued that consumption of highly processed foods, particularly edible oils and margarines, which block the oxidation processes in the cells, are responsible for the development of cancer and other degenerative diseases.** She met with great resistance from food industry giants, who were doing everything to prevent the spread of her sensational discovery. In 1952, under the influence of strong pressure from this lobby, she lost her job and was barred from the research work.

Joins Medical School at Göttingen

Opponents of Dr. Johanna blamed her that she should not treat cancer patients because she doesn't have a doctor's degree. She felt this and eventually joined medical school in Göttingen in

1955. Budwig was 47 years old at that time. She also continued her research work along with her studies. *Budwig successfully treated Prof. Martius's wife, who suffered from Breast Cancer*

One night a woman came with her small child whose arm was supposed to be amputated due to a tumor. She treated her and soon the amputation surgery was dismissed, and the child quickly did very well.

A Swiss woman came to her clinic in Göttingen. She suffered from Colon Cancer with metastasis and intestinal obstruction. Several doctors examined her, and were to be operated on Christmas Eve. On Budwig's request, she was treated by her protocol. The tumor of the colon quickly subsided. Seven weeks later, she was discharged without any detectable tumor. It is interesting that the Swiss custom officer was not ready to believe that the submitted passport belonged to same lady. Her look was so much changed! At home her daughter welcomed saying: "You look healthy, younger and more beautiful (from her book The Death of the Tumor – Vol. II).

After this, University allowed her to treat cancer patients with her oil-protein diet. She was getting miraculous results. University professors were excited with the results, but wanted that she should also include chemo and radiotherapy. She was rigid and didn't want to compromise. So she had differences and conflicts with her professors and ultimately left Göttingen (Budwig, Cancer The Problem And The Solution).

Last Destination - Dietersweiler-Freudenstadt

Eventually, she shifted to Dietersweiler-Freudenstadt, where she lived till her death. There she completed Ph.D. in Naturopathy so that she could legally treat cancer patients. She continued treating her patients in Freudenstadt. In 1968 she created unique Eldi oils for massage and enema, called Electron Differential Oils after performing precise spectroscopic measurements of the light absorption in different oils. *US pain institute has written somewhere: "What this crazy woman does with her ELDI oils, none of us manages to do via pain killers."*

Budwig conducted more than 200 lectures worldwide. Dr. Budwig was popular in the U.S. as FLAX SEED lady from Freudenstadt. She delivered her last public Lecture in Freudenstadt on March 3, 1999. On November 28, 2002, she fell down in her bathroom and got a fracture in right femur neck. She was admitted in a nursing home and ultimately died on May 19, 2003.

Budwig Protocol

The Budwig Protocol is one of the most widely followed alternative treatments for cancer and other diseases. The diet seems simple, but foods are powerful and can heal a person.

Transition Diet

The Transition diet is especially recommended for patients of liver, pancreatic or gall bladder cancers. The basic principle is that for 3 days nothing is eaten and drunk except the following written and at least three times daily warm tea (herbal teas from peppermint, rose hip, mallow or green tea) is drunk. Dr Budwig has recommended variant 1 for patients with a relatively good energy state, and variant 2 and 3 mainly for seriously ill patients.

Variant 1

Variant 1 for three days, 250 g of linomel or alternatively freshly crushed Flax seed is eaten together with the following:

Freshly pressed fruit juices without added sugar.

Freshly pressed vegetable juices such as carrot, celery juice, red beetroots and apple juice.

Chinese tea and black tea are allowed in the morning

Honey for sweetening is allowed. Just as grape juice for drinking and as a sweetener. Energetically weak patients can also consume sparkling wine and linomel.

Variant 2

For three days, oat meal cereal very hour with linomel is eaten daily with the following juices:

Freshly pressed fruit juices or freshly pressed vegetable juices such as carrot, celery juice, beetroot and apple juice.

Chinese tea and black tea are allowed in the morning.

Honey for sweetening is allowed. Just as grape juice for drinking and as a sweetener.

Energetically weak patients can also consume sparkling wine and linomel.

Variant 3

For three days, oatmeal soup with linomel is given three times a day together with the following juices:

Freshly pressed fruit juices or fruit juices without added sugar.

Freshly pressed vegetable juices such as carrot, celery juice, beetroot and apple juice.

Chinese tea and black tea are allowed in the morning.

Honey for sweetening is allowed. Just as grape juice for drinking and as a sweetener.

Energetically weak patients can also consume sparkling wine and linomel.

It is often experienced frequently that patients mixed all three variants and "nevertheless" had good results. So better you to stick to one variant. (Budwig – Cancer The Problem And The Solution 2005: p.36).

Budwig Diet

The Budwig Protocol is necessary for many diseases from cancer to type 2 diabetes and heart disease to autoimmune diseases, etc. Its purpose is to energize the cells by restoring the natural electrical potential in the cell. Many human diseases are caused by "sick cells" which have lost their normal electrical potential; generally via a lower ATP energy in the cell's mitochondria.

6:00 AM – Sauerkraut juice

A glass of sauerkraut juice consumed before breakfast every morning. It is rich in vitamins including C, enzymes and helps develop the health-promoting gut flora. Sauerkraut is cabbage that has been pickled by natural fermentation, mainly with lactobacillus bacteria. It is slightly salty, sharp and sour. Well made, it is much nicer than it sounds. You may also consume another glass of sauerkraut juice later in the day.

It interesting that sauerkraut contains right rotating lactic acids and is highly alkaline and neutralizes levo-rotating lactic acids and makes our body alkaline. That is why Marcus Porcius Cato the Elder issued a statement - Carcinomas are incurable except with the treatment with Sauerkraut.

8:00 AM Breakfast

Green or herbal tea

Start breakfast with a cup of warm herbal or green tea. Sweeten with only natural honey. You can add lemon or grape juice. Patient should take such a tea before or with Linomel Muesli. You may consume 4-5 such teas in a day.

Linomel Muesli or Oil-Protein Muesli

This should be made fresh and consumed within 15 minutes.

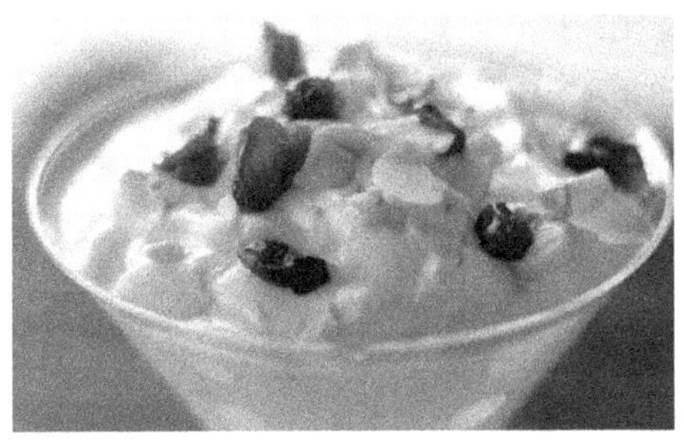

It is full of high energy pi-electrons, attract oxygen in the cells and capable of healing cell membranes. It is full of energy-rich omega-3 fats, has power to attract healing photons from sun through resonance. As "Om" is divine word and synonym of God in India. According to Hindu Mythology, the whole universe is located inside "Om", so the name Omkhand has been given to this wonderful recipe in Hindi.

Ingredients

3 Tbsp cold pressed organic Flax seed oil (FO)

100-125gm (6 Tbsp) Quark or Cottage Cheese(CC)

2 Tbsp freshly ground Flax seeds

2 Tbsp milk

1 cup fruits

¼ cup dried nuts

Natural honey

Flavorings – lemon, apple cider vinegar, cinnamon, pure cacao, natural vanilla, shredded coconut etc.

Recipe

Place 2 tablespoons Linomel or freshly ground Flax seeds in a small bowl. It is covered with raw, crushed or diced seasonal fruits depending on the season. Pour some orange or grape juice over this. Linomel Tm is a brand name and originally created and patented by Budwig. It is a cereal made from cracked Flax Seed, a small amount of honey and a little milk powder.

Then the Quark-Flax seed oil cream is prepared in as follows: First add Flax seed oil, milk and honey and blend briefly with a hand-held immersion electric blender, then gradually add the Quark in smaller portions. Blend till oil and Quark is thoroughly mixed with no separated oil. Then it is seasoned differently everyday with different flavorings such as vanilla, cinnamon or various fruits such as banana, apple, lemon, orange juice, or berries.

Use various fruits such as fresh berries, apple, cherry, orange, banana, papaya, grapes etc. Add other fresh fruit if you like, totaling ½ to 1 cup of fruit. Budwig specially advised to use berries like strawberry, blueberry, raspberry, cheery

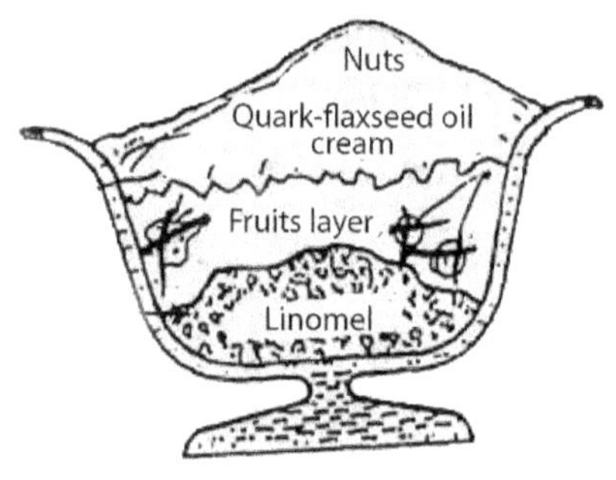

etc. because berries have ellagic acids which are strong cancer fighters.

Add organic raw nuts such as walnuts, almonds, raisins or Brazil nuts. They have sulfurated proteins, omega-3 fats and vitamins. Brazil nut is especially important because a single nut provides you with all of the selenium you need for the day. Selenium is very important to boost immune power. Peanuts are prohibited.

For variety and flavor, try natural vanilla, cinnamon, lemon juice, pure cocoa or shredded coconut.

Once blended in Budwig Cream, Quark and Flax seed oil form a new substance called lipoprotein. Lipoprotein is a water soluble complex. The Quark is rich in the sulfur-containing amino acids, methionine and cysteine. These positively charged amino acids attract the negatively charged electron clouds in fatty acid chains and exhibit a stabilizing effect on the highly unsaturated, otherwise easily oxidized fats. Thus, the amino acids protect the polyunsaturated fatty acids from the Flax seed oil against oxidation which, as a result, are able to enter the human body unchanged and with their full energy potential. The result: they are much more valuable to cells and their membranes. Consequently, one could say that Quark excels as a protector for the polyunsaturated fatty acids.

Sulfur-rich amino acids play a wealth of roles in many vital functions in our bodies. In combination with polyunsaturated fatty acids, they are important partners in regulating the uptake of oxygen and its utilization by the cell. They therefore contribute significantly to a strong immune system, healthy metabolism, and mental vitality. For many generations, people have been getting their omega-3 fatty acids from fish, vegetables, nuts, and seeds. Our health literally depends on the regular consumption of the essential omega-3 and omega-6 fatty acids, alpha-linolenic acid (ALA) and linoleic acid (LA). Our bodies require these fatty acids in order to synthesize their cell membranes as well as for a variety of metabolic processes and heal the cancer and other diseases.

Tips for making the Budwig Mixture

Follow directions properly! It is important to add things to the mixture in the right order. If you mix them in the wrong order you may lose a lot of the opportunity to convert the oil-soluble omega-3 into water soluble-omega-3.

Keep the Flax seed oil refrigerated.

Immersion blender is a must.

The mixture can be flavored differently every day by adding nuts and fruits preferably organic such as pecans, almonds or walnuts (not peanuts), banana, organic cocoa, shredded coconut, pineapple (fresh) blueberries, raspberries, cinnamon, vanilla or (freshly) squeezed fruit juice.

Consume immediately for best results.

10 AM Vegetable juice

Freshly squeezed vegetable juice from carrots, beets, celery, tomato, and radish, lemon as well as green vegetables - stinging nettle, lettuce or spinach. Apple is added to sweeten and enhance the taste. Carrot & beet juices are especially helpful to the liver and have strong cancer fighting properties. Vary vegetables. Some tasty and nutritious combinations are beet and apple juice, carrot and apple, carrot and beet, asparagus and apple, celery and apple, celery and carrot. Beet juice should not be taken alone. If taken alone it may cause red or pink urine (beeturia).

She also frequently recommended the following juices:

1. Nettle juice - Especially in the spring, Dr Budwig recommended to puree nettles with water and a lemon.

2. Radish juice - For this, a radish is first crushed and then thrown together with a lemon into the juicer. This juice is by the way durable for several days and Dr Budwig has sometimes recommended her patients to drink a small quantity of them every day.

3. Coltsfoot juice - For this juice, with the exception of the harder old rootstock, the entire remaining underground shoot is mixed with a few flowers and some milk and honey.

4. Horseradish juice - Mix 3-5 cm horseradish together with an apple and (raw) milk. Depending on the quantity of milk you can change the taste. Dr Budwig recommended this juice above all to workmen and to stimulate the appetite. Freshly pressed means, by the way, that you drink the juice within 5 minutes after pressing. In some cases, Dr Budwig prescribed a second juice 30 to 60 minutes later.

12:15 PM Lunch

Salad Platter: Salad plate with homemade cottage cheese-Flax seed mayonnaise. As salad also use: dandelion, cress, celery, tomato, cucumber, lettuce, radish, cabbage, broccoli, green horseradish and pepper.

Delicious mayo salad dressing can be prepared by mixing together 2 Tbsp (30 ml) Flax Oil, 2 Tbsp (30 ml) milk, and 2 Tbsp (30 ml) cottage cheese. Then add 2 tablespoons (30 ml) of Lemon juice (or Apple Cider Vinegar) and add 1 teaspoon (2.5 g) Mustard powder plus some herbs of your choice. Other alternative dressing can be made by mixing Flax Oil, lemon juice, Mustard and some herbs (Budwig, The Oil-Protein Diet Cookbook, 1994).

Main Course: Vegetables cooked in water, then flavored with Oleolox

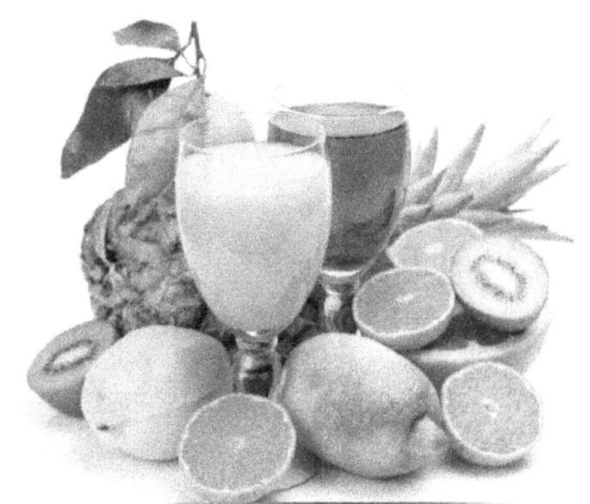

and herbs possibly with oatmeal, soy sauce, curry etc. Vegetable broth flavored with a little Oleolox and yeast flakes. As side dish for the vegetables: buckwheat, brown rice, millet or potatoes can be used. One or two slices of Ezekiel bread can be taken. Use lot of dried fruits in the main meal also.

Lunch Dessert: Cottage cheese/ Flax oil mixture served as a dessert, prepared with dry fruits and fruits such as apple, or poured over a fruit salad. You already know how to prepare it perfectly. You will find wonderful recipes for a delicious dessert in the Oil-Protein cookbook by Budwig. Please note that the dessert is **"a must"** and should definitely be eaten. So keep your main course light so you may enjoy the dessert happily.

The form of preparation as "fruit foam," "Linovita" or "red coat in the snow" (in Oil-Protein cookbook) is always welcoming for the healthy and the sick. In all the gimmicks in the preparation of the delicious desserts, one should be aware: Quark and Flaxseed give the patient immense power within a short space of time. Always fresh and beautiful, always freshly interesting, this important food for life should be for the sick and for the whole family.

3 PM Fruit juices

In the afternoon, Dr Budwig recommended different kinds of fruit juices e.g. apples, grapes, cherries, pineapples, papaya, or apricot, sparkling wine or wine - with or without Flaxseeds or with or without a few drops Flaxseed oil.

Budwig preferred papaya juice and recommended her patients to drink at least every 2 days a glass of papaya juice. The main reason for this was

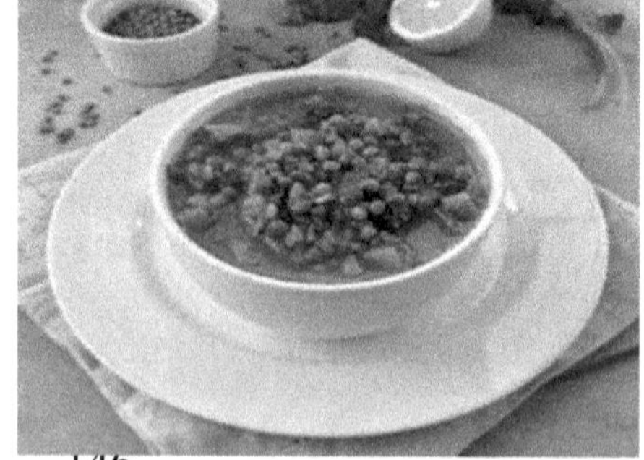

definitely the protein splitting enzyme papain.

6 PM Dinner

The evening meal should be light and served early, around 6 p.m. A warm meal may be prepared using brown rice, buckwheat or oat meal. Never consume corn or soy beans. Dishes made with buckwheat grouts are most easily tolerated and nourishing. Use only honey to sweeten. Soup or more solid dishes can be combined with a tasty sauce according to preference. Use OLEOLOX liberally also to sweet sauces and soups, making them nourishing and a richer source of energy.

8:30 PM

A glass of organic red wine may be consumed. All things are a matter of correct dosage. This glass of red wine is not a "must" program. In fact, seriously ill patients having pain and discomfort just starting on the oil-protein diet, it is recommended to serve a glass of red wine mixed with freshly ground Flax seeds to tide them over while going off pain killers (Budwig, Cancer The Problem And The Solution).

METRIC CONVERSION TABLE	
10 g = 0.35 oz	5 cc = 1 teaspoon
100 g = 3.5 oz	15 cc = 1 tablespoon
150 g = 5.25 oz	30 cc = 1 ounce
250 g = 8.8 oz	250 cc = 1 cup
454 g = 1 lb	960 cc = 1 qt
Oz = ounce lb = pound qt = quart	
Tsp = teaspoon Tbsp = tablespoon	

Precautions

Drink filtered water - Use RO (Reverse Osmosis)water for drinking, cooking and enemas.

Eat Organic Diet - Always try to eat organic food.

Dental Care –

Mercury is a Carcinogenic as well as a Poison! The root canals of dead teeth are full of bacteria that attack the liver and lymphatic system. From Amalgam fillings the mercury slowly leaks out of the filings. The ADA cleverly defends the use of amalgam in spite of the fact that there is sufficient evidence that patients with many severe problems, including psychotic episodes and fatal allergic reactions, were just cured by removing the amalgam. It is advisable to rather have a ceramic filling than be slowly poisoned by mercury. Even gold filling is dangerous; it acts as battery producing electrical current. Be informed that the effect of drugs, including poison, is dose dependant and cumulative.

Fluoride is not only toxic but it is also carcinogenic. Fluoride has never been proven to prevent tooth decay. It has been outlawed in many countries or groups of countries because the evidence is overwhelming that fluoride causes premature aging, so drink bottled water and use fluoride-free toothpaste (American Cancer Institute - 1963).

I highly recommend helping you avoid fillings in the first place. Holistic dentist recommend 3% H_2O_2 as a gargle or rinse, or making a paste using baking soda. H_2O_2 usage three times a day is advised. It is great for cleaning dentures, too.

Frying and deep frying - Frying and deep frying is not allowed to cook patient's food. Never heat any oil in the kitchen. By heating oils the wealth of high energy electrons is destroyed and Trans fats and dangerous toxic chemicals such as acrylamides are formed in the oil. Boiling

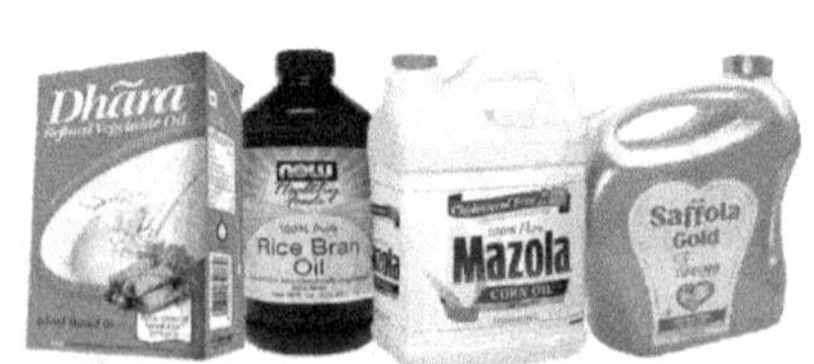

and steaming are good practices. You can fry vegetables etc. in water and add oleolox before serving. Water is the safest medium for frying, says Lothar Hirneise.

Chemo and Radio

Chemotherapy is aimed at destruction of the tumor, and it destroys many living cells, and the entire person. Anything that disturbs growth is fatal because growth is an elementary 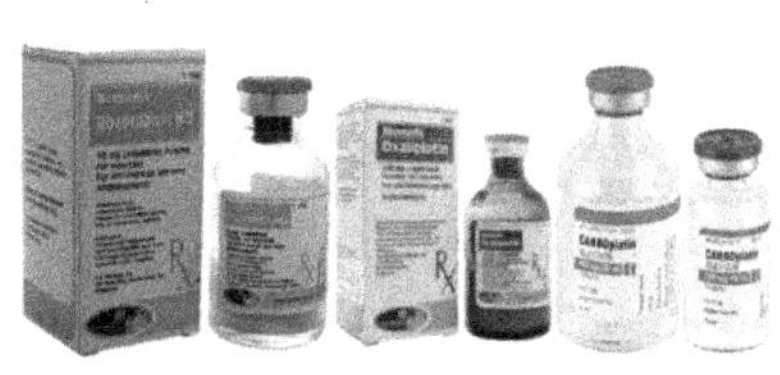 function of life. We cannot achieve something good with bad tools.

Dr. Budwig rejects Chemo and Radiation Therapy. Budwig used to say with full confidence and clarity, "My treatment targets on the real cause of cancer; it fills cancer cells with high energy pi-electrons and attracts oxygen into the cells. And cancer cells start to breathe and produce vital energy."

Man-made Supplements - With this treatment man-made antioxidants, synthetic vitamins and pain killers should not be given. The dose of anticoagulants and aspirin should be adjusted by your doctor. Dr. Budwig favors natural, herbal and homeopathy instead of man-made and synthetic supplements, vitamins and pain killers (Budwig, Cancer The Problem And The Solution).

Prohibitions of Budwig Protocol

In this protocol there are certain restrictions. They are as important as the diet itself. It is very difficult to defeat the cancer without strictly following these rules.

Sugar is strictly forbidden

Sugar, Jiggery, molasses, maple syrup and artificial sweeteners like xylitol, aspartame are not permitted. You can use only natural honey, stevia and fruit juices – all off course unprocessed.

Avoid meats, eggs and fish

Meat, fish, poultry, eggs, and butter are never allowed. Preserved meat is like a poison. It is highly processed and treated with dangerous antibiotics, preservatives and nitrates.

Stop using Hydrogenated Fat and Refined oil

You can never eat pizza, burger, fast food, fried food, biscuits etc. as they all are made by hydrogenated margarine and shortenings. Hydrogenation is a very dangerous process, used to increase shelf life of fats. In this process (oil is heated at very high temperature and hydrogen is passed through oils in presence of nickel) killing Trans fats are formed, high energy live and vital electrons are destroyed and nutrients are damaged. Hydrogenated Fats is just a dead, nutrition-less and cancer causing liquid plastic. Budwig always preached against these damaging fats. She has allowed low fat cheese, oleolox and coconut oil.

Preservatives and Processed Food

You should not eat Potato chips, soft drinks etc. which are full of preservatives. Never consume highly processed food e.g.

ready to eat packed foods, pasta, pastries, bread and soy products, tofu etc. However good quality soy souse is permitted.'

Microwave, Teflon, Aluminum and Plastic

Never cook in microwave oven. Food cooked in microwave become toxic and deformed. Also don't use aluminum, plastic, Teflon coated cookware and aluminum foils. Use stainless steel, iron, china clay or glass utensils instead.

Chemicals and pesticides are not allowed

Avoid pesticides and chemicals, even those in household products & cosmetics. Stay away from mosquito repellants, sun screen lotions and sun glasses.

Wear natural fibers

Don't wear clothes made using synthetic fiber like nylon, polyester and acrylic. Budwig put great emphasis on the fact that her patients only wore natural fabrics such as cotton or satin, since they too can influence the magnetic field of our body.

Bed

Don't use on foam pillow and mattress. She recommended horsehair mattresses. Latex mattresses are the second choice. In any case, however, you should always replace mattresses that have metal spring cores.

CRT TV and mobile phones

These emit dangerous electromagnetic radiation, so do not use them. You can watch LCD and plasma TVs.

No left over

Food should be prepared fresh and eaten soon after preparation to maximize intake of health giving electrons and enzymes (Budwig, Cancer The Problem And The Solution).

Few Desserts recipes by Dr. Budwig

Fujiya delight

Ingredients for 3 people:

250 cc grape juice, 250 cc pure currant juice,

8g agar-agar, Quark-Flaxseed oil,

Milk, honey, vanilla cream

Preparation:

Heat the grape juice till it boils, then add the currant juice, agar-agar, stirring constantly for 5 minutes, and allow to cool. Now divide this mass to 3 narrow, tall cups, which have been rinsed with cold water. It is preferable if these cups have a bottom diameter of only 3- 4 cm. Refrigerate to cool. Now mix a Quark-Flaxseed oil cream with milk, honey and vanilla. Turn the red jelly upside down onto glass plates. The Quark-Flaxseed oil cream is placed on the top so that only the upper half is covered with the Quark-Flaxseed oil cream, so that top looks like the Snow caped Mount Fujiyama.

(The beautiful hotel with a gorgeous view of the Fujiyama is called "Fujiya", hence the dessert "Fujiya".)

Linovita-in-love in wine jelly

Ingredients: for 5 people:

- 250 cc of grape juice, 250 ccm of white wine,
- 8 agar-agar, 4 tablespoons of milk,
- 8 tablespoons of Flaxseed oil, 2 teaspoons of honey,
- 200-250 g of Quark, 2 liqueur glasses
- Vodka, plum (Slibowitz) or cherry brandy or rum

Preparation:

The wine jelly is prepared by heating 250 cc of grape juice till it boils. Agar-agar is stirred with a little wine and placed in the boiling grape juice. Immediately remove from the cooking plate and add the remaining wine gradually with constant stirring. After about 5 minutes, the jelly mixture clears itself. You can now divide to approx. 5 glass bowls or champagne glasses. Immediately afterwards, mix the Quark-Flaxseed oil cream from Flaxseed oil, milk, honey and Quark. Finally, add 2 liqueur glasses of vodka or slibovitz or cherry brandy or rum into the Quark-Flaxseed oil cream. This Quark-Flaxseed oil mixture is evenly divided on the ready to-use bowls so that the Quark-Flaxseed oil cream partly sinks down in the middle. It is served after complete solidification.

Ice cream with cocoa

Ingredients:

- 3 tablespoons of Flaxseed oil, 3 tablespoons of milk,
- 1 tablespoon of honey, 100g of Quark, 100 g of hazelnuts,
- 2 tablespoons of cocoa

Preparation:

Quark, Flaxseed oil, milk and honey are mixed in the blender, then the hazelnuts are added, well blended and finally, cocoa is added to the mixture. Now pour the entire mixture into the ice-maker and place it in the fridge compartment of the refrigerator. This mixture with a nougat flavor gives the various combinations mentioned here the dark color contrasts. For very ill people these preparations are very important, especially when there is a general lack of appetite.

ELDI oils

Dr. Budwig created unique ELDI oils, called electron differential oils after performing precise spectroscopic measurements of the light absorption in different oils - specifying that the oils contained pi-electron clouds from Flax oil, wheat germ oil plus vitamin-E in its natural complex, etheric oils and sulfhydryl groups.

Dr. Johanna Budwig said, "The sun is my preferred treatment modality, as is ELDI oil, used externally to stimulate the absorption of the long-wave band of the sun. I have used ELDI oils extensively since 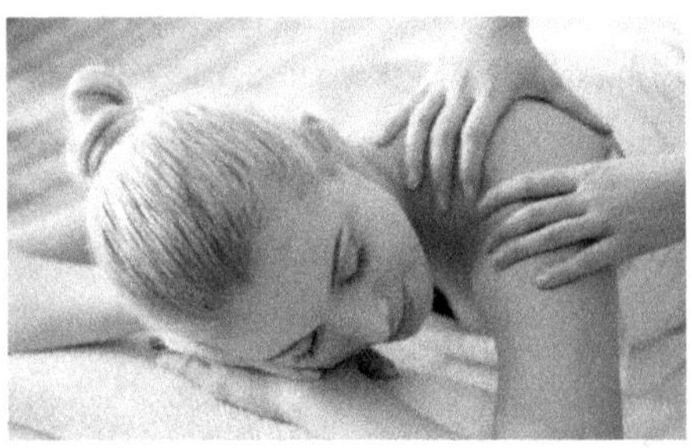 1968 for body massage as well as in the selective application of oil packs. US pain institute has written somewhere: "What this crazy woman does with her ELDI oils, none of us manages to do via pain killers." Dr. Budwig has mentioned that if ELDI oil is not available, you may use Flax oil instead.

Massage Benefits

Since ancient time massage has been part of cancer healing. Think of your lymphatics as a trash-disposal system for your body. Massage initiates lymphatic drainage, you push the trash out of your body and you're helping your immune system.

Massage therapy is sometimes the first really pleasant touch a patient is able to experience.

Massage also releases endorphins (our body's natural painkillers), stimulates lymph movement, and stretches tissues throughout the body. It's energizing, stimulating, and pretty good feeling.

ELDI oil plans:

A: For cancer patients in support of the energy level

1. Full-body rubbings in the morning

2. ELDI oil R enema with 200ml every 2-3 days

3. Wrap at the "place of the happening"

B: For energetically weak patients

1. Full-body rubbings in the morning and in the evening

2. Enema: standard plan for ELDI oil R

3. Wrap at the "place of the happening"

4. Daily liver wrap with ELDI oil sage

Additional information:

Make sure that you make once a week an (deep/high) enema with water or coffee.

If you make daily coffee enemas, then start in the morning with the coffee enema and then with the ELDI R enema, but only if your energetic level allows you to make two enemas daily. Otherwise, only make the ELDI R enema. (Oil Protein Diet by Lothar Hirneise)

ELDI oils from SENSEI (www.sensei.de) are produced in a permanent cold chain in a European oil mill and marketed under the name of Electron Differentiation Oils. There are two qualities. A 6-star organic quality and a 5-star quality, which are produced exclusively for the IOPDF (www.iopdf.com).

Cost factor ELDI oils

Again and again we hear that for reasons of cost, patients use Flax seed oil instead of ELDI oil R for an enema. Please do not do so, because Flax seed oil does not react in the same way as

ELDI oil R. Instead, use cheap ELDI oils from IOPDF or reduce the amount of oil.

Procedure –

Two times a day, i.e. morning and evening, rub ELDI Oil or Flax oil into the skin over the whole body, a bit more intensely on the shoulders, armpits and groin area (where plenty of lymphatic vessels are present) as well as the problem areas, such as the breast, stomach, liver, etc. Leave the oil on the skin for about 20 minutes and follow with a warm water shower without washing with soap. After 10 minutes take another shower, this time using a mild soap, and then relax for 15-20 minutes.

Once the body has been oiled and the ELDI Oil or Flax oil has penetrated the skin, the warm water will open the skin pores and the oil penetrates the skin more deeply. The second shower, where one washes with soap, cleanses the skin so that clothes and linen will not become overly soiled.

Oil Packs

Take a piece of cloth made of pure cotton. Cut to a size to fit the body part, such as the knee. Soak the cotton cloth with oil, place on the knee etc., cover it with a piece of polythene and wrap it up with an elastic bandage. Leave overnight. Remove in the morning and wash the knee; repeat in the evening. Keep applying the same procedure for weeks, you get good results. You also use Flax oil or castor oil for these local applications if you do not get ELDI oils . Dr Budwig generally recommended ELDI sage and should be used in the following indications:

- Tumors
- Painful skin areas
- Metastases
- Hepatic impairment and liver support
- Kidney problems

- Bladder disorders
- Intestinal cramps
- Lung disorders
- Bone disorders of all kinds

ELDI Oil Enema

Enemas are used in the Oil-Protein Diet exclusively for the energy intake and not for the purification of the intestine. Dr Budwig used to give ELDI oil or Flax oil enema to her serious patients. Budwig used to get immediate and miraculous results with the most seriously ill patients. Flax seed Oil enema also give similar results.

I recommend you to make the first enemas only with 100ml and then increase over several days to 250ml. Some patients have enemas with 500ml oil and positively reported on it. 500ml are however the absolute exception and mostly not necessary. Usually 250ml suffice.

Incidentally, smaller amounts are also easily introduced with an enema syringe instead of with an enema bucket. Enema syringes are available in sizes up to 350ml and are easy to handle.

Standard plan for ELDI oil R: Day 1 = 100ml, day 2 = 100ml, day 3 = 150ml, day 4 = 150ml, day 5 = 200ml, day 6 = 200ml and day 7 = 250ml.

From the seventh day, one remains at 250ml, and so long until the patient is significantly better. Then you can go back to 100ml - 150ml, always together with 1-2 daily whole body rubbings. (Oil Protein Diet by Lothar Hirneise)

Ingredients

- Enema pot
- Watch
- A bowl to collect oil when you are getting rid of bubbles.

- Towel and tissue
- RO filtered water
- ELDI oil or Flax oil
- Towel or Drip Stand

Procedure

Prepare a place near the toilet, so that if you can't hold the enema, you will be making a quick dash and the shorter distance is better.

Cleansing Enema with Plain water

First of all you should take a plain water enema. Purpose of this enema is cleaning of intestines. It is not a retention enema and is evacuated immediately. For this you may use 500-1000ml (2-4 cups) RO filtered water. As soon as the whole water is inside the rectum, go and sit on the commode and release the water slowly.

Take the oil enema immediately after the water enema

Use advised (above) amount of ELDI or Flax oil. The oil should be at body temperature. The best test is to dip your little finger into the oil.

Fill the oil into the enema pot. It takes at least 5 minutes for the bubbles to get out of the tube.

The enema pot should be hanged on a drip stand about 2-3 feet above your body.

You need to lubricate the nozzle and anus with Flax oil. When all is ready, lie on your right side in the fetal position. Insert the nozzle into the rectum slowly and carefully with your left hand, and un-pinch the tube.

If you feel little uncomfortable when the oil is going in, pinch the tube, wait till the feeling passes away, then continue again.

The oil is much more viscous and moves more slowly. You might need to hold the pot a bit higher to get it to run a bit quicker.

Once the oil is in, wait and hold it for about 12 minutes. After that slowly turn yourself to left side and hold oil for another 12 minutes. You may listen to music while taking enema.

When done, it is best to sit on the commode for about 15 minutes with something to read (Skelton).

Coffee Enema

Dr. Max Gerson introduced coffee enema back in the 1930s. In this enema about 500ml of coffee is pushed into rectum, this amount only reaches up to sigmoid colon. There is no loss of minerals and electrolytes in Coffee Enema because their absorption occurs well before sigmoid colon. Coffee enema is even safe for those who are allergic to coffee because it is not absorbed into the systemic circulation. You may take this enema once or twice. It has the following benefits:

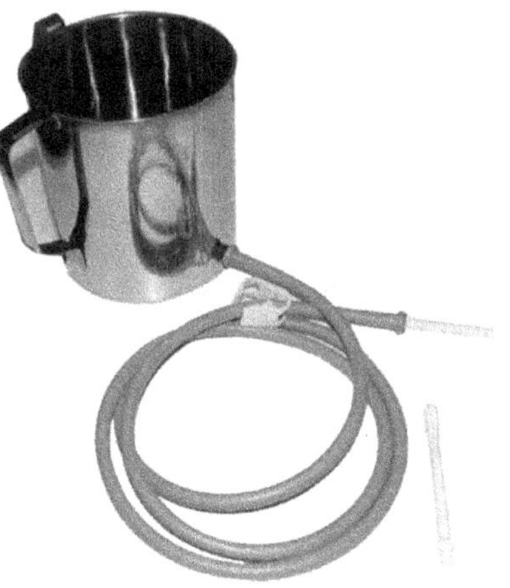

Powerful and Natural Pain Reliever

Cleansing - Coffee also acts as an astringent in the large intestine, helps cleanse the colon walls.

Toxin Elimination - The major benefit of the coffee enema is elimination of toxins through the liver. Caffeine, theophylline and theobromine dilate the blood vessels and bile ducts, stimulate the liver to discharge more bile and boost the detoxifying process into high gear and heal inflammation. Indeed, endoscopic studies confirm they increase bile output.

Stimulates Liver - Kahweol and cafestol palmitate found in coffee promote the activity of a key enzyme system called glutathione S-Transferase. This is an important mechanism in the detoxification of carcinogens, as the enzyme group is responsible for neutralizing free radicals. Coffee enema stimulates the activity of this system by 600- 700%.

Coffee Enema Procedure

This enema is retained for 12-14 minutes, during this time blood circulates in liver three times and blood is purified. Coffee enema can be given several times a day, few patients take up to seven times a day. Normally if pain is not relieved it may be taken more than one time. You should relax while taking enema; you may listen to music or read newspaper while relaxing. The best time for coffee enema is either early morning after you passed motion or during the day time.

Grind organic coffee beans. Put approx. 750ml of filtered water in a steal pan and bring it to boil. Add 2-5 heaped Tbsp coffee powder, 3 Tbsp is ideal. It is roughly 20-25grams. Let it continue to simmer for ten minutes or more and then turn off the burner. Allow it to cool down to a very comfortable, tepid temperature. Test it with your finger. It should be the same temperature as your body's temperature. Filter the coffee with fine mesh steal sieve into a jug. This is approximately 500ml.

Pour 2 cups (500ml) of coffee into the enema pot. Be sure the plastic hose is clamped tightly. Now open the clamp and grasp, but do not close the clamp on the hose. Place the enema tip in the sink. Hold up the enema bag above the tip until the coffee begins to flow out. As soon as it starts flowing, quickly close the clamp. This expels any air in the tube.

Lubricate the enema tip with a small amount of coconut oil or KY jelly. Create a comfortable and relaxing atmosphere. After a few days you will thoroughly enjoy this ritual.

Light a candle, play some light music and most importantly, make sure you are comfortable and warm. We recommend placing a pillow with a washable cover under your head and lying down on an old towel.

The position preferred is lying on your back. With the clamp closed hang the pot about 3 feet above your belly. We like to hang the enema pot on a drip stand.

Insert the tip gently into anus and open the clamp slowly. You should relax and breathe. The coffee may take a few seconds to begin flowing. If you develop a cramp, close the hose clamp, turn from side to side and take a few deep breaths. The cramp will usually pass quickly. Usually nothing happens.

When all the liquid is inside, close the clamp and remove it slowly. Retain the enema for 12- 14 minutes. You may remain lying on the floor.

After 14 minutes or so, go to the toilet and empty your gut. Take your time. Wash the enema pot and tube thoroughly with soap and water.

Take more potassium in the form of fruits and vegetable juices if you take coffee enema regularly (S.A.Wilsons.com).

Epsom bath

Detoxification of your body through bathing is an ancient remedy that anyone can perform in the comfort of your own home. Your skin is known as the third kidney, and toxins are excreted through sweating. An Epsom salt bath is thought to assist your body in eliminating toxins as well as absorbing the magnesium and nutrients that are in the water. Soaking in Epsom salt actually helps replenish the body's magnesium levels, combating hypertension. The sulfate flushes toxins and helps form proteins in brain tissue and joints. Most of all, it will leave you relaxed, refreshed and awakened. Take it once a week or as advised.

Prepare your bath

It is a 40 minutes ritual. The first 20 minutes are said to help your body remove the toxins, while the second 20 minutes are for absorbing the minerals from the water

Fill your tub with comfortably hot water. Use a chlorine filter if possible.

Add Epsom salt (Magnesium sulfate). For people 50 Kg and up, add 2 cups or more to a standard bath tub.

Then add 2 cups or more of soda bicarb. It is known for its cleansing ability and even has anti-fungal properties. It also leaves skin very soft.

Add 2-3 Tbsp ground ginger. While this step is optional, ginger can increase your heat levels, helping to sweat out more toxins. However, since it is heating the body, it may cause your skin to turn slightly red for a few minutes, so be careful with the amount you add. Depending on the capacity of your tub, anywhere from 1 Tbsp to 1/3 cup can be added (Herneise).

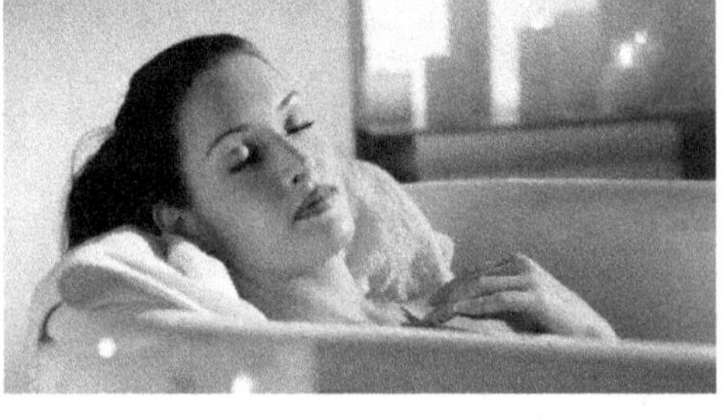

Add aromatherapy oils. Again optional, but there are many oils that will make the bath an even more pleasant and relaxing experience (such as lavender), as well as those that will assist in

the detoxification process (tea tree or eucalyptus oil). Around 20 drops is sufficient for a standard bath.

Swish all of the ingredients around in the tub, and then slip into the tub. You should start sweating within the first few minutes. If you feel too hot, start adding cold water into the tub until you cool off.

Get out of the tub slowly and carefully. Your body has been working hard and you may get lightheaded or feel weak and drained. On top of that, the salts make your tub slippery, so stand with care.

Drink plenty of water and relax in bed for a few minutes

Soda bicarb bath

Lothar Hirneise has given lot of importance to Soda bicarb bath. It is thought to assist you in eliminating toxins as well as making your body alkaline so your tumor cells may suffocate. Patient may take it once or even twice a day. Just add 2 cups of soda bicarb in your bath tub filled with warm water and relax in it for 30-40 minutes (Hirneise, 2005).

Sun Therapy

Getting an adequate amount of sunshine is a critical part of Budwig protocol. Once the body has acquired the right oil-protein balance with the Cottage Cheeseand Flax oil, the body develops better capacity to absorb the healing photons from the sun. Remember that for healing of cancer high energy photons from the sun are very important. The sunshine is important to maintain adequate vitamin-D levels in our body. Vitamin-D is a powerful antioxidant that has been linked to preventing many diseases including cancer.

Dr. Budwig's focus was on the importance of photons from the sunbeams and their interaction with vital essential fats (linoleic and linolenic acid) in our body. It is the interaction of photons from the sun and the electrons in proper food that provide the synergistic effect on healing our body. Eating the electron rich Flax oil/Cottage Cheese mixture, must be connected with adequate exposure to sunlight.

There is nothing else on earth with a higher concentration of photons of the sun's energy than man. This concentration of the sun's energy is very much energetic point for humans, with their wave eminently suitable lengths - is improved when we eat electron rich essential oils, which in turn absorbs the photons in the form of electro-magnetic waves of sunbeams.

When you eat the FO/CC mixture, your body becomes a better antenna for the photons from the sunbeam. Your body develops a better ability to absorb the energy from the sun and Transfer it to your cells to perform their vital functions. You become energized at a deep level, and when this happens cancer is healed itself.

It is red light that penetrates deeper in the tissues. In 1968 Dr. Budwig used 695 nm ruby (red) lasers light with success to radiate healthy surrounding cancer tissues in cancer patients.

How long should you take this protocol?

If all is well patient feels better and tumor start to shrink within a 3 or 4 months, if he follows treatment religiously and honestly. He may be cured in one or two years. **It is recommended that the Budwig protocol and full diet is followed for at least five years.** Even after that he should maintain healthy eating and life style.

Dr. Budwig has clearly mentioned that if you do not get the desired success, do not blame the protocol, rather try to find out your mistakes and correct them. The threshold between winning and losing is very small, and even a minor mistake can unbalance the complete healing process.

Linomel

Linomel is an invention by Dr Budwig. Freshly crushed Flax seed is mixed with honey and milk powder so that the crushed Flax seed is more stable. There is no doubt that freshly crushed Flax seed is more valuable, but also has the disadvantage that you do it yourself and clean the grinder afterwards. That is why Linomel still has an existence right. Do not buy crushed Flax seed in the shop as the chance that these contain Trans fatty acids is 100%.

Is there an alternative to Linomel?

Freshly crushed Flax seed is an alternative. This must be eaten immediately after the meal, otherwise it will oxidize.

Make your own Linomel. Mix 6 tablespoons freshly crushed Flax seed with a tablespoon of honey. Small tip: Grind the Flax seed, e.g. in a coffee grinder, and set the grinder to coarse. So it mixes better with the honey.

Daylight

Dr Budwig focused upon the importance of daylight to our health. It is not enough to absorb electrons only through food, but it is important that we feed ourselves so that our cells are able to absorb and process the light coming from the sun. The more sickly someone is, the sooner he is "in the house", which can be a catastrophic mistake. Especially when people are already in a very late stage of the illness, they are often not able to eat enough and good advice is then very difficult. In such cases, Dr Budwig advises to concentrate on the following three points:

ELDI oils as whole body rubbings and if possible as enemas

Only freshly squeezed juices and distributed as food throughout the day if possible the breakfast muesli in different variants

Stay outside as much as possible

You will experience me to explain what to do next. I have been able to see in my life how Dr Budwig's theoretical considerations work when put to practice, if indeed, if they are consistently carried out. If you could experience such a case yourself, and how quickly it can be better for a seriously ill person, you can see Dr Budwig's words in a very different light.

But other great researchers had also dealt with the subject of light long before Dr Budwig. For example, the anthroposophist Rudolf Steiner wrote, about 50 years earlier that there is a fundamental being of our material existence of the earth, of which all materiality has come only through condensation. Every matter on earth is condensed light! There is nothing in material existence, which is something else than condensed light in some form. Wherever you go and feel matter, you have condensed light everywhere. Compressed light. Matter is light by its very nature. In as much as a man is a material being, he is woven of light. Rudolf Steiner and Dr Budwig have pointed out in their writings over and over again the importance of light and that we humans are now heliotropes, which need light and use light. But I have nowhere else than with Dr Budwig so clearly and understandably read, WHY this is and above all, how the charging of the life battery works and / or what importance mainly the linolenic acid or electron clouds play. Because it is so important, I would like to repeat here again: The sicklier someone is, the more he should be in the open." (Oil-Protein Diet by Lothar Hirneise)

Disclaimer

This book is not intended to replace the advice and/or care of a qualified health care professional. Please do not try to self diagnose or self treat any disease. Seek professional help and consult your physician before making any dietary changes.

This book is not intended to provide medical advice and is sold with the understanding that the publisher and the author have neither liability nor responsibility to any person or entity with respect to loss, damage or injury caused or alleged to be caused directly or indirectly by the information contained in this book or the use of any products mentioned. Readers should not use any of the product discussed in this book without the advice of a medical profession.

The Food and Drug Administration has not approved the use of any of the natural treatments discussed in this book. This book, and the information contained herein, has not been approved by the Food and the Drug Administration.

Cancer - Cause and Cure

Based on Quantum Physics developed by Dr. Johanna Budwig

http://www.amazon.com/Cancer-Quantum-Physics-developed-Johanna-ebook/dp/B00P3Y7BYG

Book Description

******* A must have book for every cancer patient *******

This book provides an introduction of Dr. Budwig's cancer research and treatment.

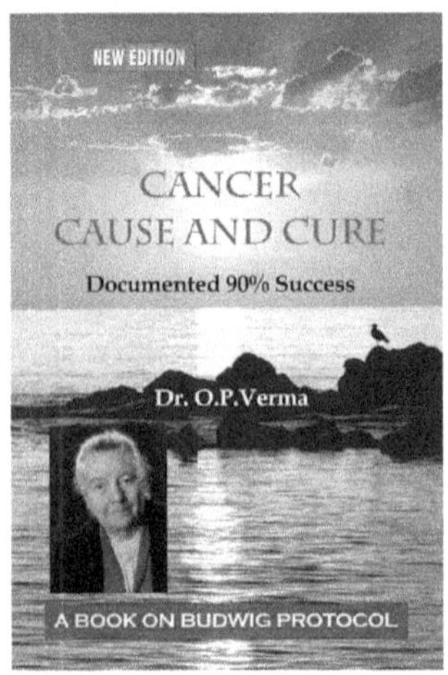

Johanna Budwig (1908-2003) was nominated for the Nobel Prize seven times. She was one of Germany's leading scientists of the 20th Century, a biochemist and cancer specialist with a special interest in essential fats.

Otto Warburg proved that prime cause of cancer oxygen-deficiency in the cells. In absence of oxygen cells ferment glucose to produce energy, lactic acid is formed as a byproduct of fermentation. He postulated that sulfur containing protein and some unknown fat is required to attract oxygen in the cell.

In 1951 Dr. Budwig developed Paper Chromatography to identify fats. With this technique she proved that electron rich highly unsaturated Linoleic and Linolenic fatty acids were the undiscovered mysterious decisive fats in respiratory enzyme function that Otto Warburg had been unable to find. She studied the electromagnetic function of pi-electrons of the linolenic acid in the membranes of the microstructure of protoplasm, for all nerve function, secretions, mitosis, as well as cell break-down. This immediately caused lot of excitement in the scientific community. New doors could open in Cancer research. Hydrogenated fats, including all Trans fatty acids were proved as respiratory poisons.

Then Budwig decided to have human trials and gave flaxseed oil and quark to cancer patients. After three months, the patients began to improve in health and strength, the yellow green substance in their blood began to disappear, tumors gradually receded and at the same time the nutrients began to rise. This way Dr. Budwig had found a cure for cancer. It was a great victory and first milestone in the battle against cancer. Her treatment protocol is based on the consumption of flax seed oil with low fat cottage cheese, raw organic diet, mild exercise, and the healing powers of the sun. She treated approx. 2500 cancer patients during a 50 year period with this protocol till her death with over 90% documented success.

She was nominated 7 times for Nobel Prize but with a condition that she will use chemotherapy and radiotherapy with her protocol. They did not want to collapse the 200 billion dollar business over night. She always refused to support the damaging chemo and radio for the sake of humanity.

The book also, describes about rare and miraculous herbs used in the treatment of Cancer like Turmeric, Black seed, Ginger, Mistle Toe, Aloe vera, Echinecea, Lobelia, Essiac Tea, Pau d'arco Tea, Dandelion, Milk Thistle.

~~**~~

Cancer Cure Is Found: Letrile is the answer

https://www.amazon.com/Cancer-Cure-Found-Laetrile-answer/dp/1797710206/

CANCER CURE IS FOUND

During 1950, a biochemist Dr. Ernest T. Krebs Jr., isolated a new vitamin from bitter apricot kernel that he called 'B-17' or 'Laetrile'. He conducted further lab animal and culture experiments to conclude that laetrile would be effective in the treatment of cancer. He proposed that cancer was caused by a deficiency of Vitamin B 17 (Laetrile, Amygdaline). Laetrile is a concentrated and purified form of vitamin B17. After a lot of research, he had finally developed a specific protocol to treat cancer. Laetrile Therapy combines Laetrile with nutritional supplements and a healthy diet to create a potent treatment that fights cancer cells while helping to strengthen the body's immune system.

Vitamin B-17, which is present in several different foods, consists of a locked substance which comprises two units' glucose, one unit benzaldehyde and one unit cyanide. When B17 comes in contact with a cancer cell it is unlocked by a hormone found only in the cancer cell, and becomes a lethal chemical bomb which destroys the cancer cell. Healthy cells do not cause breakdown of B17. Cancer is unknown to people living in areas with food products rich in B-17, and the population lives to a remarkably high age. Apparently nature has provided us

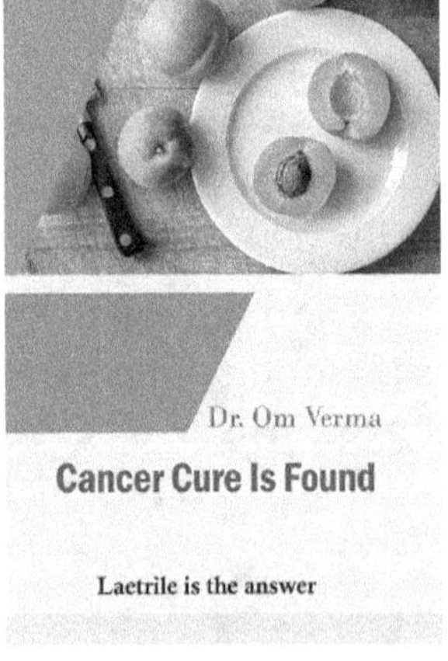

with an ingenious defense against cancer, and it is an ordinary nutrient in our food. These are, amongst others nuts, seeds, vegetables, and in particular apricot kernels.

At present, patients listen or read a lot about Laetrile treatment, but usually they don't get precise and to the point information about what are the exact components of this protocol, where to get Laetrile injections and supplements, what to take, what not to take, what are the doses, how long to take the treatment, what diet they have to follow, etc. In this book, I have explained the protocol in detail proposed by Dr. Krebs. I have given every minute detail about Laetrile, other nutritional supplements and diet in this book. After reading this book patients can buy Laetrile injections, tablets and other nutritional supplements from the reliable sources (given in the book) and conduct the treatment under the supervision of their family doctor. Dr. Philip E. Binzel was personally trained by Dr. Ernest T. Kreb Jr. about everything of this treatment. Dr. Binzel had been using Laetrile therapy in the treatment of cancer patients since the mid 1970s. His record of success was astounding. Testimonies of his patients are also included in this book.